Recovering from your broken tibia

A practical guide to healing from intramedullary nail surgery, from one patient to another.

Sara Bussandri

Recovering from your broken tibia. A practical guide to healing from intramedullary nail surgery, from one patient to another.

Copyright © 2018 Sara Bussandri

ISBN 978-1986445597

Published by Sara Bussandri 2018.

Contents

PART THREE: APPENDIX

Disclaimer

Any information contained in this book is **for general educational and informational purposes only**. **It is not intended or otherwise implied to be medical advice**. **You should always consult your doctor or other health-care professional to determine the appropriateness of this information for your own situation, or if you have any questions regarding a medical condition or treatment plan**.

Foreword

This book specifically covers **fractures of the tibia that require the insertion of a tibial intramedullary (IM) nail or rod (also known as a Küntscher nail) through a surgical procedure**. It is largely based on my personal experience of having an IM nail inserted into my right tibia in 2016 in the UK (you can find my full story in the Appendix). However, care has been taken to add information from research and experiences others have shared with me that may be helpful in your case.

It aims to inform **adult patients** about the **recovery and healing process** from this type of fracture and specific surgery, with particular focus on the **practicalities and adaptations required during this time, including any related physical, mental and emotional implications**. However, some sections of this book could also be useful for:

- Anyone who finds themselves using crutches or wearing a plaster cast due to a different type of injury.

- Anyone caring for a child who experienced a similar injury and surgery, although surgical options and recovery times may be considerably different.

- Anyone experiencing a fracture of their femur (upper leg) who had a femoral nail/rod inserted in their broken bone.

- Anyone looking for natural ways (including diet and lifestyle changes) to aid the healing process after a bone fracture.

For the purpose of this book, it is assumed that you have no other fractures, injuries or existing medical conditions that may or may not be a result of the traumatic event that caused the fracture of your tibia. **No advice from this book should ever replace medical advice.**

Of course, it goes without saying that no two tibial fractures or surgeries are the same. Everyone's situation, circumstances and health conditions are different, so you may find parts of this book that are not applicable to you.

I would like to also take this opportunity to thank the NHS and in particular all the staff at West Middlesex hospital (UK) for the excellent medical care I received during my hospital stay.

Who is this book for?

This book was written for someone who has broken his or her tibia in such a way that it requires the **surgical insertion of an intramedullary nail into the medullary cavity of the bone**, or for someone who cares for a person who has undergone this procedure.

If you have broken your leg and are reading this, you have all my sympathy. I hope you find reassurance and support in the information contained within these pages. It was written taking into consideration everything I wish I had known when I was in hospital that first night with a cast on my leg, waiting for surgery and wondering how myself and my family would cope for five or six months in that situation.

I would also like to acknowledge that whatever happened that caused you to break your leg was a traumatic event. Your tibia is a very strong bone and it requires a lot of force to break it, which is why you're probably under the care of the Trauma and Orthopaedic team. You may have been doing something very mundane in a relatively safe environment (such as climbing the stairs at home, like me), playing sport or enjoying a leisure activity, or you might have been involved in a serious accident. Of course, you might have other injuries or there might be other people who are hurt or involved too. Whatever the case may be, this was not planned.

Regardless of what you were doing when you had your accident, you could not have known that you would end up badly injured. There is no denying that this unfortunate event will impact and shape your immediate future as well as the future of the people around you. You undoubtedly had other plans that now need to adapt and change. This book will help you during that process.

Why this book?

When I broke my leg in September 2016 and was told that it would take five or six months for me to be able to 'get back to normal,' I found myself not really able to grasp the concept. I just could not comprehend how it would take so long for my bone to heal, especially when I had been told I was being offered surgery to help it heal better and quicker. At that point in time I found myself suddenly bedridden, heavily medicated and unable to understand what my life in the immediate future would look like.

Of course the doctors and surgeons who cared for me were very open to answering all the questions I had, but their focus at that point was mainly on fixing my leg. Their concern was to address the fracture and give me the best chance to recover and heal correctly. But I needed to know more! I wanted to understand how I would care for myself. What would the next few months look like for my family and me? Would I always be in this much pain? How long would I be bedridden for? How long would it take for my leg to fully heal? When would I be able to walk, run or drive again? Would I need help around the house? Could I do anything to speed up my recovery? These were not questions I felt I could ask my surgeon, but who else could give me the answers I needed?

As I'm sure you know, resorting to Google when it comes to a medical condition can take you down a very different and sometimes dark route. There is a lot of medical literature available online, but not all of it is immediately accessible if, like me, you don't have any medical training. The terms can be very technical and obscure, and it may not be very productive for you to go through the results of several clinical trials. And let's not lie to each other – you may even stumble across things that totally terrify you! I know I did.

I wrote this book to try to answer all the questions I had that first night in hospital and describe the things I learnt during my recovery. With my immediate plans out of the window and our family dynamics suddenly turned upside down, I was determined to find out how to make my situation work for us. Over time, I was able to answer all the questions I had around the practicalities of my day-to-day life and the emotional and mental impact of my fracture. Documenting my thoughts on my blog mindyourmamma.com and reading up to find ways to help my body cope with the effects of the injury and surgery massively helped me through this process.

My desire is to be able to help anyone who is going through the same experience and make them feel a little more in-the-know and in control of their situation. What I wish is for someone who finds themselves with a broken tibia to read this book while they're in hospital waiting for surgery. And I hope it will be a good companion for them while they look for information, advice and reassurance on what's to come.

Part One: Trauma and Surgery

1. Your fracture

I will not spend a huge amount of time on this section because if you have found this book, unfortunately you have already fractured your tibia or are close to someone who has. You may feel that you have enough information about your broken bone and the surgical options that have been recommended to you, as your doctors would have already filled you in. However, I will include it for completeness and for those of you who may find yourselves waiting in their local A&E department/Emergency Room and looking for more information on their fracture and the medical terms you've probably just heard for the very first time. If this part of the book isn't relevant to where you are on your recovery journey, feel free to jump straight to Part Two, which deals with your recovery.

What is a tibial fracture?

We have two long bones in our lower leg – the tibia and the fibula. The tibia is the larger bone of the two, and the one we can feel at the front of our shin between the knee and the ankle. When it comes to our lower legs, the tibia is the one that supports our weight. You may have heard your doctor or specialist call it a 'weight-bearing' bone.

The fibula is a lot thinner and is non-weight-bearing. It is located in the lower leg to the side of the tibia, and is also called the calf bone. It serves the important function of stabilising the tibia, but it does not support our weight. Because it typically takes a major force to break a long bone such as the tibia, other injuries often occur at the same time, and when the tibia breaks it is very common for the fibula to break as well.

The tibia can break in several ways, and the severity often depends on the amount of force that caused the injury. For example, a 'tibial shaft fracture' is one that occurs along the length of the tibia.

Once your lower leg has been X-rayed, your doctor should be able to tell which type of tibial fracture you have and whether the surgical insertion of an intramedullary (IM) nail is the recommended and best option in your specific circumstances. Typically, open (compound) fractures or fractures with large degrees of displacement or that are unstable will be good candidates for IM nailing.

Common types of fractures

Your doctor will probably have told you what type of fracture you have, or you may have seen this in your notes. They will have probably gone through your X-rays with you and given you an explanation of what has happened to your bone, but you can find more information in the following pages.

These are the most common types of fractures:

Stable fracture – this type of fracture occurs when the part where the bone has broken remains in place. In other words, the broken ends of the bones are still aligned. In a stable fracture the bones usually stay in place during healing.

Displaced fracture – when a bone breaks and is displaced, the broken ends are separated and no longer line up. This is also called an **unstable fracture** and often requires surgery to put the pieces back together before healing can start.

Transverse fracture – this type of break has a horizontal fracture line. The fracture can be unstable, especially if the fibula is also broken. This means that the fracture can also be displaced (see above) and therefore might require surgery.

Oblique fracture – a break that has an angled pattern and is typically unstable. If an oblique fracture is initially stable or minimally displaced, over time it can become more out of place.

Spiral fracture – this is caused by a twisting force. The result is a spiral-shaped fracture line around the bone, like a staircase. Spiral fractures can be displaced or stable, depending on how much force caused the break. I experienced a closed, stable, spiral fracture, and you can read more about my personal circumstances in the Appendix if you're interested.

Comminuted fracture – so-called because the bone has shattered into two or more pieces, and the fracture is considered very unstable.

Open or compound fracture – when broken bones penetrate through the skin it is called open or compound. Open fractures often involve much more damage to the surrounding muscles, tendons and ligaments. They have a higher risk of complications and take a longer time to heal. As circumstances around the open and compound fractures can be varied or specific, they will not be covered in this book.

Closed fracture – contrary to an open or compound fracture, in the closed fracture the broken bones have not penetrated the skin. However, it is possible for internal soft tissues to be damaged.

2. First aid and emergency treatment of your fracture

Signs and symptoms of a broken leg

If you're currently in the A&E department/Emergency Room of your hospital with a suspected broken leg, you may experience some or all of these symptoms:

- Swelling and/or bruising.

- Pain in the injured area that gets worse when the area is moved or pressure is applied.

- Loss of function in the injured area – when you try to move your leg or your foot it simply does not respond in the way that you want.

- Deformity of the injured area – this is especially true and obvious in case of a displaced fracture, where the bone might be visible under the skin, and in cases of an open fracture where the bone may have penetrated through the skin.

- You may (or may not) have heard a snap when the bone fractured and you might (or might not) hear a grinding noise when the area is moved.

- You may be feeling faint, dizzy or sick.

Of course, depending on the traumatic event that caused your leg to break you may have suffered other injuries and may be experiencing other symptoms as a result of those. If the fracture has just occurred, you may not be aware of any of these symptoms yet, as levels of adrenalin in your body are still very high at this time. If your fracture is open or compound and the bone has exited the skin, you may have also lost blood and be in a state of haemorrhagic shock. Therefore you might be experiencing further symptoms, such as low blood pressure, rapid and shallow breathing or a weak pulse etc., and you may need to be treated for shock.

First aid treatment

You may be past this stage already, but I will include this information for completeness in case it is still relevant for anyone reading.

- When a broken leg is suspected, you should always try to immobilise the injured area.

- If the bone has penetrated through the skin, it is important to try to stop any bleeding.

- You may notice that if you tried to use your leg or foot you were unable to do so. If this happened, listen to what your body is telling you and avoid putting any weight on your leg.

- A broken bone **always** requires medical attention. The first thing that needs to happen is for the extent of your injury to be determined, so you will need to have your leg X-rayed. It is only after this happens that the best treatment for you can be determined. So if you haven't already, you should get yourself to the nearest hospital as soon as possible. Remember that you should continue to keep your leg immobilised, so if you're on your own you will need to call an ambulance.

X-rays

An X-ray will be performed in the radiology department of your nearest hospital or emergency centre. X-ray procedures are normally painless, but with a broken bone it may not be the most pleasant experience. While the X-ray technicians place your leg in different positions to perform the necessary tests, it is important that you continue to do your best to keep your leg stable. The pain will be persistent, but when your leg is maintained in a straight and stable position, you will feel that the discomfort is minimised. This also reduces the risk of creating any further injuries, such as the bone penetrating the skin if it hasn't already.

Please remember that while the X-ray technicians will do their very best to take your pain into account, they do need to obtain a number of different views of your leg so that a full diagnosis can be made for you, so they will need to move you and your leg a number of times in order to do so. Take your time during the process and ask them to slow things down and ask to take a quick break if you need to. The experience will be painful, but it's necessary to help you get better.

Did you know?

- If you are wearing any jewellery, you might be asked to remove it.

- If you are pregnant, or if there is a chance that you could be pregnant, you should inform your doctor and X-ray technician(s). Measures can be taken to protect your baby from the radiation involved, but a risk is always present. If you are pregnant, whether you go ahead with the X-ray examination despite the risks to your unborn baby will ultimately be your choice, but in the case of a broken leg, your healthcare professional might insist you do indeed go ahead as it would be otherwise very difficult to make an accurate diagnosis without being able to visualise your fracture.

The diagnosis

Once your doctor has had a chance to examine your X-rays, they should be able to make a diagnosis. This is when you will be informed about the type and extent of your fracture and the recommended treatment.

If your tibia is fractured, and the surgical insertion of a tibial intramedullary (IM) nail has been recommended to you in your specific circumstances, **you should also be informed at this point about the pros and cons (including the risks) of the surgery, as well as any alternative options available to you.** You may be feeling emotional and confused right now, but it's important that you – or someone who is with you – ask any questions you may have. You will probably be required to sign a consent form to say that you agree to the surgery being performed, although this may also happen later just before the surgery is ready to begin.

Temporary plaster cast

If you have experienced an open fracture and lost a lot of blood as a result, you may be treated for haemorrhagic shock and be immediately taken to theatre for surgery. This is because your wound needs to be cleaned up and irrigated (washed out) as soon as possible.

If your tibial fracture is closed and surgery cannot be performed on the day of your accident, in order to avoid your fracture becoming unstable and creating more damage you may be required to wear a temporary cast, also known as a 'back slab.'

While you are lying on your back, various layers of plaster will be wrapped and moulded around your leg. To stabilise your tibia, it is very likely that your ankle will need to be included in the plaster cast. If so, it will be gently positioned at a 90-degree angle before it's also wrapped in plaster. Your toes will typically be outside of the cast.

Depending on where on your tibia the fracture is, you may require an above-the-knee-cast to add further stability to the bone. If this is the case, your knee will be placed at a 30-degree angle while supported by cushions or blankets to make you more comfortable.

This procedure will most likely be performed by one or more doctors, with the assistance of a nurse. You may experience pain while the plaster cast is applied to your leg. If you do, it's important to let your doctor know so they can help you manage your pain with medication, if you're okay with that. You may be offered paracetamol, Entonox (also known as nitrous oxide or 'gas and air') or morphine in the form of an injection.

Once the temporary plaster cast has been applied, you might be taken back to the X-ray (or clinical imaging) department to ensure the fragments of your bone have been aligned correctly. Effectively, your fracture has to be immobilised in the best possible position to avoid further damage and minimise pain.

Your broken fibula

If you've broken your tibia, chances are your fibula is also broken. You may have been told your fibula is broken but may have also noticed that not much emphasis is being put on this fact. The fibula is non-weight-bearing, meaning that its role is to stabilise the tibia rather than supporting your body weight when you stand up or walk. Unless your fracture is really serious, in most cases the fibula heals by itself within approximately six weeks. Had you just broken your fibula and not your tibia, you may even be told you can walk on it while it heals. However, it may be that you have also experienced a serious fracture of your fibula, and you may require a plate (and screws) to be fitted around the bone while your tibia is being attended to.

3. Waiting for your surgery

Unless you required immediate surgery, once your leg has been placed in a temporary cast (or back slab), you are likely to be admitted into hospital while you wait for your surgery to be performed. If your fracture was closed and you didn't have further complications, there is a chance you may be sent home. This can only happen if your doctor is happy that the fracture is sufficiently immobilised through the temporary cast. If this is the case, the hospital will contact you to schedule your surgery.

The emotional impact

Something that is often overlooked is the emotional side of your experience. It is likely that, while being treated in your local hospital, you're receiving the best possible level of medical and professional care. Your fracture is being looked after by a number of very experienced professionals, and if you're staying in hospital you can be sure that you're in the best place you can be.

But we need to remember you've recently experienced a traumatic event of various degrees of severity. As a bare minimum, you're likely to be a little (or very) shaken. You may not even be consciously aware or able to verbalise this yet, so it's important that anyone caring for you or supporting you through this event is able to take how you feel into account.

Whatever it was that caused your tibia to fracture, it was something unexpected, sudden and unplanned. You had not set off on that day knowing that something like this would happen. Breaking a bone isn't something you can ever be prepared for!

Once immediate medical care has been provided and your fracture has been stabilised, the realisation you've now broken your leg will hit you. Whatever plans you had for that day, week or even upcoming months are now likely to change. Whether it's business or personal (such as a holiday, wedding, or social gathering), this is likely to create some worries or heightened emotions.

Whether at home or in hospital, you'll be immobilised for a few days while you wait for your surgery. You'll most likely be bedridden and unable to do things for yourself, and that can be both frustrating and plain hard to deal with if you're on your own.

Depending on your own personal circumstances, this fracture can have a considerable (yet hopefully temporary) impact on your life and the lives of the people around you. It's completely acceptable for you to feel overwhelmed and upset by the situation at least some of the time, and definitely immediately after your injury happened.

It may sound easier said than done, but if you can, try to:

- Talk to someone about how you're feeling.

- Be patient and kind to yourself during this difficult time.

- Be positive – yes, this has happened to you and yes it's awful, but the best thing you can do for yourself and those around you is to put all your efforts into getting better as quickly as possible. Having a positive attitude and outlook will definitely make the next few months easier for you.

We'll cover more on this in section 6.

Observations and medications

If you were admitted into hospital while waiting for your surgery, you may now be transferred to a ward. Be prepared for your nurses to 'take your observations' quite often – your blood pressure, temperature, and oxygenation level readings will be monitored at regular intervals during the day and night.

Your nurses will also help to manage your pain by offering painkillers. Remember that with any medical procedure or intervention, ultimately the choice as to whether to take anything is yours. If you feel you don't need any medications for your pain, you don't have to take any.

If you routinely take any medications or have any allergies, your nurses will ensure you receive the relevant drugs at the right time.

Blood clots – risk and prevention

Once in hospital, you are likely to be bedridden for a few days. This is because until your surgery has been performed it is not advised that you attempt to walk on your temporary cast. The fact you just suffered a significant injury and trauma, coupled with the temporary inability to walk, puts you at an **increased risk of developing a blood clot**. Blood clots may form in one of the deep veins of the body, and it is estimated that about two-thirds of all cases occur during or after a hospital stay.

To protect you against this risk, you may be offered daily doses of **blood thinners** (also known as anticoagulants). These reduce the chance of developing a blood clot by slightly thinning your blood. The blood thinner most commonly used is called heparin, which is given by injection. Ask your local healthcare professional for any specific information that applies to your country.

In order to further reduce the risk of you developing a blood clot, you may also be asked to wear an **anti-embolism stocking** on your 'healthy' leg. They work by compressing your leg gently. You're advised to wear them day and night (whether in hospital or at home) until you return to your normal level of mobility. Ideally, you should remove your stocking daily to have a wash and check for any skin problems or soreness, but you should not be without it for longer than about 30 minutes.

Keeping your leg elevated

If you were admitted to hospital, you will have likely been moved around on a wheel bed or in a wheelchair. Your porter and nurses will help you transfer onto your hospital bed and get you comfortable on it.

You should **keep your leg elevated above heart level at all times** to reduce swelling and prevent inflammation. In order to ensure that your leg remains elevated, your nurses might help you prop your cast up with a few pillows. This may require a bit of trial and error at first – if your leg is left in a painful or uncomfortable position, make sure you ask for help to reposition it in such a way that no tension is applied to your broken bone.

Using the toilet

Unless you've been provided with crutches and have been shown how to use them safely – which is unlikely to have happened at this early stage of your treatment – you will not be able to get up from your bed when you need the toilet. The safest and easiest option for the time being might be for you to use a bedpan or urinal. This is so that you don't have to move or lower your leg, which can be uncomfortable and even painful. You'll probably require help with this at first as the temporary plaster cast is quite heavy, and especially if it goes above your knee as this means you can't bend it and may struggle to move.

You may find using a bedpan or urinal a bit tricky and embarrassing at first if you haven't used one before. Try to remember that your nurses are there to help. They understand your situation, as you're not the first (and unfortunately won't be the last) person they help with this.

An alternative to using a bedpan or urinal is a commode chair. This is similar to a wheelchair with an opening and bowl in the middle (a bit like a portable toilet). If one is available and you feel otherwise well — and your injuries allow it — you can ask your nurses to help you sit on the commode chair. It's likely you'll still need to keep your leg elevated and on top of the bed, so you may require help and assistance with this. Alternatively, if you're confident enough to do so you may even be able to ask your nurses to help you move onto a wheelchair so you can go and use the hospital bathroom. Be mindful of the fact that a nurse may still need to be with you inside the room to help you with your leg.

As complicated as this may sound, do remember that this is a temporary situation — try to do whatever feels comfortable and easier for your leg. The hardest thing is probably going to be accepting that you now need help. Getting assistance with going to the toilet certainly isn't something you had planned to do, so try to be patient and welcome any help that's being offered. Your nurses understand what you're going through and are there to help and keep you safe and comfortable.

Washing

Using the toilet is not the only thing you're struggling to do for yourself right now. You're likely to be bedridden for the time being, so it may not be possible for you to access the hospital showers or wash room.

Every morning, your nurses should provide you with a bowl of warm soapy water so you can have a wash. If you need any help they will be available to assist you, but if you do want and need some privacy, you can also try to do as much as you can by yourself, or ask your partner to help if possible.

Remember that initially, because of your plaster cast (and especially if you have one that goes above the knee that prevents you from bending your leg), you may also need some help when changing underwear.

Sleeping and resting

Sleeping in hospitals is notoriously difficult! First of all, unless you have your own private room you're likely to be on a ward with a few other patients. They might have different conditions and needs, which might require constant attendance during the night. Remember that your nurses will continue to come and check on you, take your observations and offer you any medications you may be taking (including painkillers) at regular intervals. Although the lights will be dimmed or switched off in the night (with only emergency lights being left on), your nurses will need to walk into the ward regularly to assist you and the other patients, so do expect some disturbance.

But that's not all. In the first few nights after your fracture, you're likely to experience various degrees of pain and discomfort from your injury. You are, after all, hurt, finding yourself in an unfamiliar and unplanned situation, bedridden, wearing a heavy plaster cast on your leg, possibly unable to move and it can be quite hard for you to get comfortable and sleep properly. With your leg still propped up and unable to bend it or move it to the side, you'll be forced to sleep on your back without being able to change positions throughout the night. This can be hard for most of us, so be prepared to sleep in short naps. As difficult as this may sound, do try to rest as much as you can. Your body is facing a 'crisis' at the moment, and you need all the rest you can get.

Fasting and IV

While you're waiting for your surgery, you may be required to fast in preparation for the operation. This means that you will not be allowed to take anything by mouth ('nil by mouth') – i.e. no food or drink – for a few hours before surgery.

To ensure that you stay hydrated, a method called intravenous (IV) rehydration is likely to be used. Effectively, sterile fluids are injected directly into your veins. This fluid solution generally contains water with salt or sugar added to it, but this might vary depending on your individual needs and circumstances. The fluid will be kept in a bag raised up above your head. For this to work, a short, small plastic tube will be inserted directly into your vein using a needle. Access is normally obtained through a vein in your arm or hand. You may experience a little discomfort when the needle is first inserted, but you should feel relatively comfortable when the tube is then covered with a little cap and a plaster when not in use. Having the tube means your nurses can access it whenever they need it without having to insert another needle each time.

The same access point may also be used to give you other drugs, such as antibiotics if you need them, for example. The plastic tube may feel a bit uncomfortable when you move your hand or arm, and it's important that you do try to stay still when the IV fluid is on, as when the tube bends, the fluid may not be able to go through. Your nurses will be able to assist you if the flow stops (and you find the machine starts beeping!)

4. The surgery

Intramedullary nail surgery (or intramedullary rod fixation) explained

If the surgical insertion of an intramedullary (IM) nail or rod (also known as an 'inter-locking nail') has been recommended, a **specially designed metal rod will be surgically inserted into the 'medullary cavity' of your tibia** through a guide wire passed across the fracture inside the bone. The medullary cavity (or 'medulla') is the innermost part or central cavity of the bone shaft. It is also known as the 'marrow cavity,' as this is where bone marrow is found.

This type of surgical procedure was introduced in the late 1930s to treat fractures both in the femur and the tibia. Although similarities might be found with patients who have had a nail inserted in their femur (femoral nail), this book focuses on tibial IM nails only, i.e. a nail that is inserted into the marrow cavity of someone's tibia to treat a fracture of the tibia, not the femur.

The main objective of the nail is to keep the bone into an optimal position and alignment to allow it to heal properly and quickly. Some of the benefits of having the nail inserted are:

- The risk of non-healing (or 'non-union') of the bone is reduced.

- The patient should be able to return to normal functions quicker.

- The nail is meant to share the load with the bone, thus allowing partial (if not total) weight-bearing within a few weeks from the fracture and before the bone has fully healed.

Please remember that whether you can or cannot bear weight on your leg after your surgery entirely depends on your own specific fracture and circumstances. You should always ask your doctor whether you can put *any* weight on your leg after your surgery. Putting too much weight on your injured leg too soon can compromise your recovery and even cause further damage to your bone.

In order to give the nail more stability within the bone shaft and obtain proper alignment of the bone fragments, special screws (known as interlocking screws) are also used. At times, when additional stability is required additional plates or external braces might also be used to keep the bone or bone fragments in place or to give the fracture more stability. This completely depends on your individual circumstances. With severe open fractures or very unstable fractures, for example, a frame outside the leg may be required to hold the bone in the correct position and to allow access to any wounds caused by the broken bone.

Why have I been offered this surgery?

It is likely that this surgical procedure is offered to you if:

- You have better chances to heal quickly by having this surgery than without.
- You are healthy and present no further risks or complications that may make the surgery not suitable for your circumstances.

The alternative to this procedure is for you to wear a plaster cast for a much longer period of time (often close to six months or more). This obviously entails a much longer period of complete inactivity and can therefore have a negative impact on potentially healthy joints, such as the ankle and (sometimes) the knee, as these would be immobilised by the plaster cast.

Another reason why this surgical procedure may be the best option for you is that correct alignment and healing through immobilisation with a plaster cast are not guaranteed, especially for fractures where the bone ends are not fully aligned (which is often the case in displaced fractures). This is also known as risk of 'non-union.'

The good news is that after you fully recover from surgery, you should be able to return to a certain degree of mobility far sooner than you would without the surgery, and even better, it is more likely that your bone will heal correctly, thus preventing further issues for you both immediately as well as later on in life. After the surgery, you may be required to wear a plaster cast to increase stability or to wear an orthopaedic or protective boot. However, chances are that you may not require either of these at all.

Risks

Intramedullary nail surgery does of course carry risks. **Always ask your surgeon about any alternative options before agreeing to have surgery**. There will be risks either way, and you should be empowered to make an informed decision. The risks include:

- Non-union – even with the nail inserted, there is a risk that the bone fragments may not heal, especially if they cannot be re-aligned or re-positioned optimally during surgery.

- The nail selected and inserted by your surgeon may be too long for your tibia. It may end up interfering with soft tissues and tendons, thus causing pain.

- Damage to the patellar tendon, which is the ligament that connects the bottom of the kneecap (patella) to the top of the tibia.

- Blood clots.

- Infection.

- Nerve injury.

- Vascular injury.

- Risks associated with having a general anaesthetic.

Potential side effects

There are also common side effects associated with this type of surgery, which include:

- Persistent knee pain.

- Local nerve damage.

- Tenderness where the screws, plates or incisions are located.

- Cold intolerance.

- Dull, constant ache.

While these symptoms appear in some patients, they don't affect everyone. Some patients with knee pain, for example, report that things improved when the hardware was eventually removed. In such cases the pain was potentially caused by the nail being too long and affecting soft tissues and tendons in the knee area. For other patients, the removal of the nail didn't seem to have an impact in improving the knee pain, which could be caused by other factors. It's important you discuss all these risks and potential side effects with your surgeon in order to make an informed choice.

Did you know?

IM nails come in different lengths and diameters to fit most tibia bones. It is down to the surgeons performing the operation to select the most appropriate one for the individual patient and their specific fracture. Tibial IM nails can have a diameter of 9–10mm or more, (depending on the individual), weigh around 57 grams (2 oz.) and are often made of titanium.

Further reading

If you want to find out more about the other types of surgery or interventions available for tibial fractures, including their pros and cons, the article 'Adult Lower Leg Fractures' on loptonline.com has more information on this. You can also find a lot more information on how the surgery is performed on the website wheelsonline.com (search for 'Tibial Fractures: Techniques of IM Nailing'). However, this site is aimed at a medical audience. It contains terms that could be unclear, but also very graphic images of actual surgery being performed. Don't watch if you think this might upset you any further!

The day of your surgery

On the day of your surgery, your surgeon or team of surgeons are likely to come and introduce themselves to you. This is a chance for them to explain how they're planning to address the procedure. For example, they may explain whether they're planning to use any plates or if they have any concerns about any aspects of your injury, etc.

Although you may still be in state of shock and disbelief, this is your chance to ask them any questions or address any doubts you may have. This is also your chance to really understand the risks associated with the surgery, so be sure to ask the question. **You want to be aware of all the risks specific to you, your fracture and your individual circumstances**. If possible, ask your partner or a relative to help you with this if you feel you need to. Also, remember to ask for any alternative solutions. What would happen if you didn't consent to the surgery?

If your fracture was open (i.e. the bone penetrated the skin), secondary surgery procedures may also be required in your case and these will be discussed with you.

General anaesthetic

Once the orthopaedics are ready for you, you will be taken just outside the operating theatre (pre-op room). The surgery will be carried out under general anaesthetic unless there's a specific reason why this is not recommended for you (for example, should you be pregnant). If general anaesthetic isn't an option, alternative options will be discussed. At this point you'll meet your anaesthetists, i.e. the doctors responsible for giving you the correct dosage of drugs that will keep you asleep during your surgery.

The doctors will check your notes and medical history and ask you some basic questions about your health and lifestyle (including any pre-existing conditions, any medications you are taking or any allergies, etc.) This is so that they can determine which anaesthetic is best suited for you.

When ready, they will give you specific medications that are used to send you into a state of deep sleep. This will be done either via liquid that is injected straight into your veins through a cannula (a thin plastic tube that feeds into your vein, usually sited on the back of your hand and potentially the same one used for your IV drips), or via gas, which you breathe in through a mask.

The anaesthetic drugs should take effect very quickly – you might start to feel light-headed at first and then become unconscious within a minute or so. After this point, you will not be aware of what happens before or during the surgery, and you will not feel any pain while the surgery is carried out. Your anaesthetist(s) will remain with you throughout the procedure and make sure you stay in a controlled state of unconsciousness. They will also give you painkilling medicine through your veins so that you're relatively comfortable when you wake up.

For more information about general anaesthesia, including side effects, complications and risks, you can read more on the nhs.uk website ('General anaesthesia').

Post-surgery recovery

Once your surgery has been completed you will be woken up in a separate room, sometimes referred to as the 'recovery room.' Here a nurse will make sure that you're awake and take your observations for a while until they're satisfied you're well enough to return to the ward.

When you wake up after the surgery, you're likely to experience some pain and discomfort in your lower leg. Your anaesthetist will have already given you some strong pain medication (most probably morphine, provided that you're not allergic to it) towards the end of your surgery.

If you can have morphine, your nurse may install a machine by the side of your bed and connect it to the cannula on the back of your hand or arm (the one used for the IV drip). This allows for morphine to be released straight into your veins at regular intervals in order to keep your pain under control. Even though you're likely to be feeling a little groggy, you'll be given a remote that you can use to release the right amount of morphine into your body when you need it. Don't worry about doing this too much or too often – the button on the remote will become temporarily unresponsive if it's too soon for you to receive your next dose. Once sufficient time has passed the button will become functional again.

Depending on the circumstances of your fracture, your leg may be plaster cast-free after your surgery but covered by a bandage and dressing. Alternatively, external braces may have been fitted or your leg may be in a new cast.

Once your nurse is happy with your post-operation observations, you'll be taken back to the ward.

Part Two:
Your Recovery

5. The first 48 hours

For the first couple of days after surgery you're likely to feel quite weak. Assuming that the surgery went well, you may (or may not) experience some of the side effects of the general anaesthetic, including:

- Feeling sick and vomiting.
- Shivering and feeling cold.
- Confusion and temporary memory loss.
- Bladder problems.
- Dizziness.
- Bruising and soreness in the area where your cannula was inserted, especially if the same one has now been used for a few days since you were admitted into hospital.
- Sore throat (especially if a tube was inserted in your throat to help you breathe during surgery).

You will not be able to get up from your bed for the first few hours, so at this stage you'll most likely continue to use a bedpan, urinal or commode chair after your surgery. See section 3 for more information on this.

Pain management

Just like after you first got injured, it's important that your pain is managed during the first few hours and days following your surgery. If you're in the UK, you may come across a Pain

Management Doctor, whose role is to devise a plan that the nurses can follow to manage and lower your pain. You may have a healthcare professional with an equivalent role in other countries.

For the first night (or two) you may be offered intravenous morphine, i.e. morphine that goes straight into your veins through a cannula. Other painkillers you might be offered are paracetamol, ibuprofen and codeine. Always remember to ask why a particular type of medication is being recommended to you and what the side effects are (especially if you don't normally take these particular medications). If you feel comfortable pain-wise, be mindful of the fact that you can refuse to take any medication should you want to.

Having said that, you're likely to find the first couple of days quite hard. When the effects of the anaesthetic drugs start to wear off, you may be feeling a lot of pain and discomfort at the fracture site but also in your knee and ankle. The pain you're in, coupled with the side effects of the anaesthesia, the medications you're taking, the reality of what's happened and what's ahead starting to kick in means you'll probably find that the first couple of days after surgery will be the hardest. But things will get better!

Antibiotics

Following your surgery, it's very likely that you will be offered antibiotics to prevent any infections. Your doctor or nurses will be able to advise you as to which type of antibiotics they recommend.

In order for the medication to be most effective, you may be given the antibiotics intravenously, i.e. via the cannula that you probably already have in your hand or arm and which was used for the anaesthetic drugs as well. You might experience some discomfort during the injection as the liquid is pushed through your veins. Alternatively, you might be able to take antibiotics as tablets by mouth.

Blood thinners (anticoagulants)

You'll probably continue to take 'blood thinners,' also known as anticoagulants (see more in section 3), for the duration of your hospital stay and for a while after being discharged (approximately two weeks, but this will depend on your individual circumstances). Although blood thinners don't actually thin the blood, they do help to reduce the risk of developing a blood clot.

There are several types of anticoagulants that you can take orally in the form of tablets or capsules. Your doctor will be able to advise you on the best one for you. As per section 3, you may be offered a medication called heparin, which is given by injection (normally in the thigh or stomach). When you're staying in hospital your nurse will continue to do this for you, and before you're discharged they'll show you (or a family member) how to safely give the injection.

If you're in the UK you may also be provided with a special type of bin to safely dispose of used needles – this is called a sharps disposal bin, and your nurse or doctor should be able to explain how you arrange for its collection once you're finished using it.

If you want to find out more about anticoagulant drugs, why you take them, how they work and what side effects they have, you can read more on nhs.uk ('Anticoagulants').

Non-weight bearing, light-touch weight-bearing or partial weight-bearing?

Depending on your individual fracture, after your surgery your doctor should be able to advise you on whether you're allowed to put any weight on your injured leg. **It's very important that you know how much weight (if any) you can put on your leg before you attempt getting off your bed, as putting too much weight on your fractured tibia too soon could compromise your recovery.**

You'll probably be in one of the following situations:

- You cannot put ANY weight on your leg – **non-weight-bearing (NWB)**.
- You can put very minimal weight on your leg, i.e. just enough to balance yourself while you walk with crutches – **light-touch weight-bearing (LTWB)**.
- You can put partial weight on your leg – **partial weight-bearing (PWB)**.

- You can put full weight on your leg – **full weight-bearing (FWB).**

In most cases you will not be able to put full weight on your leg (FWB) until your leg has healed, but more on that later.

Your doctor will be able to give you more details and information about weight bearing, so make sure you ask them any questions you may have and are very clear on what you can and cannot do. There might be individual exceptions, but the bottom line is that **even with the insertion of an IM nail, you will not be able to put full weight on your fractured tibia until it has completely healed or re-united. This may take an average of 24 weeks, depending on your individual circumstances and type of fracture**.

If you've been told you're either non-weight-bearing or light-touch weight-bearing, please be aware that this will change over time. As the broken parts of your tibia knit back together, you'll be able to increase the weight you can put on your leg. Your doctor will monitor you and advise you on this as you attend your post-op check-ups.

Getting out of bed

Soon after your surgery, when you have recovered from the effects of the anaesthetic, you may be visited by a physiotherapist. If you're strong enough and don't have any injuries in your arms, you'll be advised to start using crutches.

If you're in the UK, you may be able to borrow a pair of crutches from the NHS for free if they are available. Your physiotherapist will adjust the crutches for you and teach you how to use them safely. In the UK, you will not be discharged from hospital until your physiotherapist is satisfied that you've learnt how to use the crutches safely, so you will be shown and have a chance to practise things like:

- How to get up from your bed or from a chair.
- How to sit back down from a standing position.
- How to walk with crutches.
- How to go up and down stairs.

You may need a few sessions with the physiotherapist in order to learn how to use the crutches confidently. Don't forget that you've been bedridden for a few days by now. You've also just had surgery, so it's likely you may be feeling weak and dizzy. This is completely normal and will pass. Your physiotherapist will continue to help you until you are confident enough. Be kind to yourself and try not to put yourself under too much pressure if you can't successfully use your crutches straight away.

As you get more confident on your crutches, you may start to be able to get up occasionally to walk to the bathroom or sit on a chair by the side of your bed or in the visiting room, for example. Don't be surprised if you're still feeling a little faint initially when you try to stand up – just take your time and make sure you're safe while still getting used to the crutches. And remember **not to put more weight than you should on your broken leg**.

Getting discharged

You'll probably be discharged from the hospital a couple of days after your surgery, depending on how well you are and on whether you've successfully learnt how to safely use your crutches.

Before you are discharged, your nurse will probably:

- Change your dressing and provide you with enough bandages so that you can either change your dressing yourself, or explain where and how often you should get it changed. If you're in the UK, you may be advised to book an appointment with the nurse at your GP practice to have the dressing changed. If not, do ask your nurses or doctors about this.

- Explain which medicines you should continue to take, how often and for how long. You may be provided with the medications to take home with you or be given prescriptions to get your own from a pharmacy.

- If you're having heparin injections (see section 3 and 5), they will show you or a family member how to give them. Some hospitals may lend you a sharps disposal bin for the used needles.
- Provide you with your hospital notes.
- Provide you with the details of your first follow-up appointment with the orthopaedist or surgeon.
- Answer any outstanding questions you may have.

If you're in the UK, a team called Occupational Therapy may provide you with equipment you can use at home that will make it easier for you to go about your daily routines while you can't put full weight on your leg.

For example, I was able to borrow the following:

- A pair of crutches.
- A raised toilet seat.
- A toilet frame.
- An adjustable-height chair.

More on this later in section 9.

When you're ready to leave, ensure you have appropriate, comfortable footwear for your non-injured ('good') leg (you won't need any for your injured leg). You may need some help with leaving the hospital. Consider asking someone if they can collect you and help you with your things (especially if you have equipment to take home) and with your leg. Even though you may not be wearing a plaster cast, you may still have difficulties in bending and moving your leg at this point, as it will be swollen and sore from the surgery.

6. What will it really be like? Your questions answered

How long will it take for my tibia fracture to heal?

Healing time will be specific to the type of fracture you experienced and will depend on your age, general health and lifestyle choices. Everyone heals differently and at different speed. Here are some facts that may help:

- A minor fracture can take around six–eight weeks to heal.
- **Some tibial shaft fractures heal within four months.**
- **However, many may take approximately six months (an average of 24 weeks) or longer to heal.** This is particularly true with open fractures and fractures in patients who may not be in full health.

When we're talking about recovery and healing, it's important to understand the difference between a fully healed tibia that can bear your full weight and a healing bone that can bear at least some of your weight. As you heal, you'll be able to put progressively more weight onto your leg, and as this happens your recovery will start to feel much easier.

Your doctor will inform you about how much weight you can put on your leg and how much you should move it. Remember to stick to this advice. See section 5 for an explanation of the terms non-weight-bearing, light-touch weight-bearing, partial weight-bearing and full weight-bearing.

How long you're non-weight-bearing for (i.e. you can't put any weight on your leg), if this applies to you, also depends on where on your tibia the fracture was. You could be looking at as little as six–eight weeks, but also as long as eight–twelve weeks for more serious fractures.

During this time, while your leg cannot support your full weight you will need to use crutches, a wheelchair or some other form of mobility aide (more on this later). Remember that if you've been provided with crutches or any other mobility equipment, you should be shown how to safely use it.

How will I be feeling?

- If you're not wearing a plaster cast following your surgery, you might be feeling quite vulnerable in the first few days or weeks. You could accidentally bump your leg into things at home or anyone you live with might bump into you.

- Your leg will still be swollen, bruised and sore from the fracture but also from the surgery, so expect the bruising to take its course and heal in its own time.

- During the first few days, you may feel a rush of blood and throbbing pain whenever you lower your injured leg onto the floor, ready to stand up from sitting or lying down. If that happens, and you find it really uncomfortable, consider resting the leg on the floor for a few minutes before you try to get up.

- Remember that you recently had a general anaesthetic and it will take a while for your body to fully recover from its effects.

- You've probably been taking opiates (morphine, for example) and are most likely still on very strong painkillers (such as codeine, if this has been prescribed to you). These can cause drowsiness and side effects, and you may be feeling quite tired and 'not yourself' for a while still.

- Bear in mind that you've been bedridden and indoors for a few days by now. You probably hardly got out of bed at all and didn't get any sunlight for quite some time. These things matter! You may be feeling dizzy and weak when you try to stand up and that's to be expected. This will pass in a few days.

- You're not yet used to walking on crutches, and they can take some getting used to. You may find yourself getting frustrated and feeling extremely limited in your movements and in what you can do, but things will get better as you get used to your crutches and recover from your injury and surgery.

- You may still be **feeling shocked and agitated** (for example having flashbacks) thinking about the way you got hurt, especially if it was a particularly traumatic accident.

- You may be feeling **sad or worried**. Breaking your leg and suddenly finding yourself in this situation will obviously have immediate repercussions on your life and the people around you. You may be worried about how you will care for yourself, let alone your children or pets if you have any. Or you may be thinking about how you will cope with not being able to work or drive and the potential loss of income. If this is the case for you, unless you have insurance it could be a real concern. Try to discuss this with your doctor – they may be able to inform you about any local organisations that can offer advice or support.

- You may be experiencing a certain degree of **anxiety** in relation to your injury or accident. If you're not yet familiar with it, try to find out about **mindfulness meditation**. Through very simple and accessible breathing exercises, you should be able to relax and feel calmer when anxious feelings start to creep up on you. Also, through a technique called 'body scan,' you'll be able to focus on the sensations in your body and understand where you may be feeling tension or discomfort. If this sounds totally alien to you, consider downloading an app like Aware, Calm or Headspace, for example, to get an idea of how mindfulness can help; alternatively, YouTube has lots of resources that might be able to help you.

Anxiety and fear are normal feelings following a traumatic event. Your body has been through a huge shock, and it's only normal to feel worried about anything similar happening to you again. For example, later on in your recovery you may find yourself uncomfortable in large crowds when people get too close to your injured leg. Or you may feel very anxious if you return to the place or activity that caused your injury in the first place. Time, coupled with the practice of mindfulness, can really help you with this. For more information on how mindfulness helped me, you can read 'Injury-induced anxiety – the scary feeling of feeling scared' or 'How mindfulness can help heal a physical injury' over on my blog mindyourmamma.com. However, if you experience any excessive, uncontrollable bouts of anxiety that you feel you cannot manage on your own, be sure to speak to your doctor.

- At times, you may even find yourself feeling **angry and frustrated**. You may feel like you're **letting people down**, especially if you have others depending on you, such as an elderly parent or young children, for example. When looking at your own situation right now you may be **feeling stuck and powerless. Don't underestimate these feelings**. This may perhaps sound silly to you right now, but your injury could have an impact on your mental health, and while this is completely normal, it is also preventable. If you can, try to talk to someone you trust. And if you ever feel that negative emotions may be getting on top of you, consider asking for professional help and support. Right now, having a positive attitude and outlook despite everything that's happened can really help with your recovery. And while being optimistic may be the last thing you want to try to do (it's not easy!), it really has the potential to help you heal faster.

- If you have any children, you may be worried about how your injury will affect them. This may sound harsh and a little oversimplified, but children do adjust. Depending on how old they are, it's important you explain what is happening to you in a way that they can understand, so reassure and encourage them to address any feelings and emotions they may go through as a result of your injury. Children (especially young children) are naturally more mindful than us adults and more interested in the present, so they are often able to adjust really quickly once they know what 'the deal' is.

My children were seven, four and two at the time of my injury. They knew I was hurt and needed crutches to get about. They accepted that as a simple fact, without any judgement or worry attached to it. They would make sure my crutches were never too far away from me, or when they fell over (crutches do fall over a lot) they were the ones picking them up for me. I can honestly say that during those months, they definitely showed a lot more patience and empathy.

Will it always be this painful?

The good news is that no, it won't always be this painful. To manage the pain, in the first few days and weeks you may be prescribed painkillers such as paracetamol or codeine. This may depend on you where you are, your doctor's preferences, and your individual circumstances, so be sure to **always follow medical advice and instructions when taking pain management medications**.

While the pain will get better after the first few days and weeks, it's important to know that the pain and discomfort is caused by the natural inflammation that occurred in your body following the accident. The inflammation is an essential component of the fracture healing process, and inhibiting that process through medication (although it works for the pain) means we can effectively create a delay in the healing process if certain drugs are used. For example, non-steroidal anti-inflammatory drugs (NSAIDs) such as aspirin or ibuprofen aren't recommended for fracture pain relief. Acceptable alternatives are medications that contain acetaminophen and codeine. Once you feel the pain starts to reduce and you can manage for longer without medications, do consider cutting down. The good news is that pain can also be reduced by increasing the consumption of anti-inflammatory nutrients (through diet or supplementation). See section 10.1 for more information on this.

Will I be able to sleep?

For the first few days or weeks, you may find that the only way to sleep is on your back. This is because you'll need to keep your leg elevated on a pillow (or two) and might still struggle to turn it independently. It will probably hurt when you turn it or lay it on its side, so you won't have a lot of freedom to move around when you sleep. This may mean you could be feeling quite uncomfortable at night, both because of the pain in your leg but also because of the position you're forced to sleep in. Over time, this might start to affect your back.

However, the good news is that after a while (approximately a couple of weeks after the injury), you should be able to comfortably turn over in bed and sleep on your side. If you're not wearing a cast, you may find you need to keep your leg fully supported by using a pillow in between your shins when lying on your side. If not, you may feel some tension or discomfort around the fracture site.

When the bone becomes strong enough this soreness will start to disappear. Your injured leg muscles will also get stronger, and you'll find you're progressively able to move around in bed from one side to the other without having to support the leg with a pillow. Until then, try to be patient. The first few days and couple of weeks will definitely be the hardest, but you'll soon adapt and find a way or position(s) to sleep and rest comfortably.

My leg is bruised and swollen – is this normal?

Once again, your doctor or nurses will have informed you about your personal circumstances when you were discharged from hospital. **If you're ever in doubt or notice any changes (worsening) in your injured leg, be sure to contact your doctor.**

You can expect your leg to be swollen and bruised for a few days or weeks. The bruise is caused by the swelling under the skin, and if you've ever observed one before you'll know it takes a few days or weeks for it to fully heal, and it will change colour a few times in the process. You'll notice the bruise on your leg go through different shades until the blood is finally reabsorbed and it is no longer visible.

In order to minimise swelling, try the following:

- **Keep your leg elevated.** When you sit down, you can have your injured leg resting on a stool with a cushion, for example. Or if you're on the sofa or in bed, consider lying down and propping your leg up with a few cushions or pillows. It won't make for comfortable sleeping or resting, but it will help the healing process. Ideally, you want the leg to be above the level of your heart.

- **Move your ankle and knee** if you can and as much as you're comfortable with (as long as you don't have any further injuries or are not in a plaster cast). See section 10.2 for more information on this.

- **Apply an ice pack** on your injured leg to help with the bruising and swelling and to provide some temporary comfort. You can continue to do this at regular intervals for several weeks or even months after your surgery.

- **Massage your leg.** As long as this doesn't interfere with your wounds or surgery incisions, use your hands, a lacrosse ball or a roller to massage your leg. This is one of the most common ways to help blood rush to the affected area and start the healing process.

What about my wounds?

Even though you may not have had any wounds as part of your original injury, you do now. Your lower leg might be wrapped up in sterile bandages, or you may have adhesive dressing covering the incisions made during the surgery. These wounds will take a few weeks to heal.

You'll probably have a longer incision along your knee (this is the location where the nail was inserted), and smaller incisions where the interlocking screws were attached if any were used. If so, these are likely to be just under your knee (on the inner side of your leg) and by your ankle. If your injury required you to have additional metal plates inserted for increased stability (for example around the tibia or fibula) you may also have further incisions.

Depending on what your surgeon used, you may have dissolvable stitches, stitches that need removing or staples. Your doctor will explain what you need to do (and when) to get any stitches or staples removed if this applies to you.

Your doctor or nurse will have advised you to keep your wounds **clean and covered**, especially for the first couple of weeks, to help prevent infections and scarring. Ensure that you follow your doctor's instruction on how to care for your injury.

You may have also been given a spare dressing and shown how to use it, so you can change it yourself if your wounds ooze or are a bit wet, or you notice the gauze getting grubby. Alternatively, you may be encouraged to visit your local doctor or nurse so that they can change the dressing for you.

If you notice something unusual about your wounds, you should contact your doctor or emergency services. For example, look out for:

- Redness, increased pain or yellow-green pus, especially if combined with a high fever. These could be signs of infection.

- Black edges around the area.

- Bleeding at the injury site.

- Pain at the wound that will not go away.

- A wound that has come open, or the stitches or staples have come out too soon.

At some point you'll be able to leave your wounds uncovered. Don't be tempted to pick or scratch at the scab, as this can delay healing and cause scarring.

Try to be mindful of your wounds (and, later on, your scars), as an incision on the knee in particular may continue to be quite sensitive. Avoid kneeling on it, as you may find this too uncomfortable or even painful. If you wear jeans or particularly thick trousers you may even find that the act of bending your knee and the material rubbing on your scars creates some discomfort. If you shave your legs, make sure your wounds remain dry while they're healing and don't apply any shaving cream or product directly on the wounds while they're still open.

My skin is very dry. Is this normal?

As your wounds and skin heal, you may find that the skin on your leg becomes extremely dry to the point that it may even start to flake off. If this happens to you, it's nothing to worry about. It's likely to have been caused by the swelling in your leg, which effectively stretched the skin, causing cells to separate and flake off. Once the swelling has gone down, this should improve. To manage it, make sure you drink plenty of water, exfoliate your skin regularly and moisturise your leg, being careful of your wounds if they're still not completely healed. **You shouldn't use moisturiser or any products on open skin**. If you're unsure, do check with your doctor or nurse.

Will I need a wheelchair?

You may be wondering whether using a wheelchair, at least temporarily, could be easier and safer than using crutches. This is totally up to you. Having used one in the past when I was 13 years old and had broken my other leg, I did consider getting one following my recent injury. However, I then decided against it as I thought it would be really hard to move around in the house. Some areas would be inaccessible to me and I'd still need crutches for steps, stairs and access to the bathroom, for example.

If you decide to get a wheelchair, consider getting one that's lightweight, relatively narrow and foldable. Don't forget this is only a temporary adjustment, and if it makes you feel safer, more comfortable or if it makes life at all easier for you (for example when going out), it could be a good option. You can borrow one, hire one or buy your own and perhaps sell it once you no longer need it. Whatever you decide to do, make sure you do your research in advance, understand how big or heavy the wheelchair is, whether it'll go through your doorways or fit in the boot of your car, etc.

Instead of crutches, you could also consider using a walking frame (wheeled or non-wheeled). These may offer you more stability if you feel too frail or insecure on crutches.

You may have also seen that knee walkers are available, but these will not be an option for you because they rely on you resting your knee on a padded surface and supporting your weight through that, and you can't do that because of the incision on your knee.

Finally, if you're looking for safer options that will allow you to be more independent when outdoors while you're non-weight-bearing, you can look into electric-powered wheelchairs or mobility scooters. These are similar to an electric-powered wheelchair but designed more like a motor scooter. Depending on where you are in the world, you may be eligible to hire one for free or alternatively hire or purchase one yourself, should you decide to.

Will I be able to drive?

Although legislation may vary by country and might not be widely accessible or explicit, **safety should always come first**. Not just *your* safety, but the safety of everyone else on the road too, so driving with a broken leg is probably one of the things you shouldn't consider doing!

Having said that, a quick internet search pointed me to forums where people admitted getting behind the wheel of automatic cars with a broken left leg (in a cast even!). I am no expert and cannot comment on the legality of this, but let's just say that to be on the safe side, you should as a minimum:

- **Check with your specialist, doctor or healthcare professional whether you are allowed to drive.** If you've broken your right leg, you probably physically won't be able to until you can put full weight on your leg.
- As your leg starts to heal, speak to your car insurance provider to discuss your specific circumstances before you get behind the wheel.

Having broken my right leg, I drove for the first time 21 weeks after my injury, *after* being discharged from the orthopaedics department. At my 15-week check, my specialist told me I'd be able to drive anything between four to eight weeks from then, depending on when I felt confident enough to put all my weight onto my leg to successfully perform an emergency brake.

However, he also specifically told me **NOT to drive until I had been discharged from their care**. His reasoning being that should I be involved in an accident when under specialist care for a broken leg, my car insurance could be invalidated. In all honesty, I took his word for it and didn't check whether this piece of information was correct, but driving with a broken right leg was physically impossible for me for the first few months. And it certainly wasn't worth the risk for the sake of waiting a few more weeks. Your situation may be different, so make sure you always check with your specialist and, if in doubt, with your car insurance provider.

Can I fly?

Once again, this will vary depending on your individual circumstances, but I am aware of people who were injured while abroad and flew back to their home country as soon as their injuries were stable so that they could have their surgery there. Others had the surgery abroad and were flown back home as soon as they could travel after the surgery.

Otherwise, if you're well enough and **your doctor gives you the go-ahead**, you should be able to fly within a couple of weeks of your surgery if you need to. Do check with your doctor or insurance company as to whether you are required to take any paperwork with you when you fly.

Also, don't forget that flying (especially long-haul) increases the risk of DVT (deep vein thrombosis) and you may experience some swelling or discomfort in your injured leg. To minimise the ill effects of flying, it's advisable to wear compression stockings and gently exercise your leg as much as you can during the flight.

And if you're worried about the hardware in your leg setting off the metal detector during the security checks, this never seems to happen, but you're bound to have the guilty look on your face when you go through so it might be best to tell airport staff!

7. Getting around on crutches

If you haven't used crutches before, they can be quite tricky to handle at first. Hopefully you will have been shown how to safely use your crutches before you left the hospital. In the UK, you will not be discharged unless and until your physiotherapist is happy you know what you're doing with them. This is important because **crutches aren't the safest piece of equipment you can use, and you can hurt yourself if you use them incorrectly**. For example, you're not just at risk of slipping or falling, but if you don't handle your crutches correctly when getting up or sitting down, you risk hurting your wrists and arms.

Types of crutches

Depending on where you are in the world, and on the nature of your injury, you may be using one of two types of crutches:

- Underarm crutches.
- Elbow crutches.

What you're about to read is relevant for both types. However, if you're using the armpit ones make sure they don't actually come into your armpits when you're walking. You can rest on them, but if you put your weight onto the crutches through your armpits as you walk, I'm told it will hurt. Plus, your hands are going to go numb and you definitely don't want that!

Underarm crutches have hand grips (the bits you hold on to) and elbow crutches have cuffs. These are the bits you slide your arms into. **Do ask your physiotherapist or healthcare professional to help you with the specific type of crutches you are using if you're unsure.** Is there anything in particular you should be aware of in your circumstances?

Walking on crutches

In order to walk safely on crutches, you should place both of them onto the floor, making sure the rubber tip has a good grip, then place your weight onto your arms and crutches and swing forward with your good leg. Remember that **when walking, crutches always stay with your injured leg.** Place your crutches on the floor away from your feet; in other words, make sure you have a wider support base and go for a smooth movement, not a hop. Also, try to **aim for small steps** – huge strides aren't necessary and can throw you off-balance.

- If you're **non-weight-bearing**, it's probably safer for you to keep your injured leg away from the floor altogether.

- If you're **light-touch weight-bearing**, you can gently rest your injured foot on the floor to help your balance.

- It's only when you're **partial weight-bearing** that you can put your injured foot onto the floor to help you with walking a little, **being sure not to put too much weight onto the leg too soon.**

If and when you are advised to put partial weight on your leg, you may start to use one crutch instead of two. See section 11 for walking with one crutch.

Getting up and sitting down

When you're trying to get up from sitting, you should slide to the edge of your seat, place your crutches together side by side on one side and grab them both by the hand grips with one hand. Make sure the rubber foot (or crutch tip) at the end is firmly on the floor, then put your weight on your non-injured (or 'good') leg using both your arms and push yourself up. Only once you're in a standing position and are confident enough with your balance should you slide your arms inside the cuffs. You can watch the video 'From sitting to standing using crutches' by Kaiser Permanente Santa Rosa on YouTube if you haven't been shown how to get up with your crutches or if you can't remember how to do it.

When you need to sit down, reverse the process. First things first, ensure the place you're about to sit on is stationary. Trying to sit on a wheelie chair might not a great option when you're still learning! Start by having your back towards the surface that you are going to be sitting on (i.e. a chair). Be sure you have your balance, and only then take your arms out of the cuffs, place both crutches on one side (holding them by the hand grips with one hand) and place the other hand on the surface you'll be sitting on. If your injured leg is non-weight-bearing, make sure to put all your weight on your good leg and your hands and arms when you sit back down. The video I mentioned above will show how to safely sit down as well.

Expect sitting down and getting up to be a bit tricky at first, especially if you're trying to sit on or get up from a low surface. Chairs and stools tend to be easier to manage than sofas, beds or toilets, especially at first. As a general rule, the lower the surface, the harder it may feel to sit down or get up again. If possible, to make your trips to the bathroom a little easier on yourself use a toilet frame and a raised toilet seat (more on that in section 9).

Getting in and out of the car (as a passenger)

If you're sitting in a car (as a passenger), be mindful about the fact that car seats can be quite low. So make sure that, as you would with a chair or any other surface, you have your back to the seat before letting go of your crutches. Then put them to the side, hold on to the seat, lower yourself onto the car seat, swing your legs in first and then bring your crutches in. You may be more comfortable doing this the other way, depending on which side you're sitting on. The only thing to be really careful of is the door – don't hold on to it, as it can move or close! Hold on to the seat instead. For more information on driving, see section 6.

Getting up and down from the floor

I'd advise that you avoid sitting or lying on the floor, at least initially if you can. A few days or weeks after your surgery, you may want to do some upper-body exercises that don't impact your injured leg. Sometimes lowering yourself onto the floor can become a necessity, especially if you're home alone and have dropped your phone or TV remote under the sofa!

So, if you really need to lower yourself onto the floor, make sure you do this next to a firm and steady surface. Get yourself next to this surface, move both crutches to the side (holding on to them with one hand) and use the crutches and the sturdy surface to lower yourself down onto your **good** knee. You will not be able to put your injured knee on the floor for a long while – even though your knee wasn't originally injured, this is where the incision for the surgery was made. It will be a really long time until it no longer feels uncomfortable to kneel down on your 'bad' knee (we're talking months or possibly years).

When you need to get up again, get onto your good knee, grab hold of your crutches with one hand and the steady surface with the other, and use your upper body and the muscles in your good leg to push yourself up.

Going up and down stairs

Going up and down the stairs with an injured leg and a pair of crutches can be quite intimidating at first, but chances are you do have steps or stairs at home, so it's important you know how to handle them safely.

Stairs with a handrail

If the stairs have a handrail, hold onto it with one hand. You'll be holding both your crutches with the other hand by the hand grip. How? One crutch will be pointing down, with the rubber tip firmly placed on the step, and the other crutch will be perpendicular (i.e. at a 90-degree angle) to the first crutch, pointing towards the top of the stairs if you're going up. If the stairs have a handrail, you won't be needing both crutches while walking up the stairs (as one hand will be holding onto the rail), but you still need to take the second crutch upstairs because you will need it once you reach the top. This method may sound dangerous at first, but you do get used to it with practice.

So, to go up the stairs pull yourself up with the arm that's on the handrail, place your full weight onto your good leg and your one crutch. You proceed up by having the crutch you're using behind your injured leg. So your injured leg goes up one step first (without putting weight on it), then you place your full weight onto your good leg and the crutch (which are on the same step now), and you push your good leg onto the next step. You do this by placing all your weight on your arms through the handrail and the crutch.

Once you reach the top of the stairs, you take the crutch you were holding but not using with the hand that was holding on to the rail, and then start walking as you normally would.

To go down the stairs you reverse the process. While you hold both crutches in the same side with one hand by the hand grips (as you did while going up), you now **put the good leg one step down first** and you follow with the injured leg and foot.

Although this may sound really confusing when you first read it, a good way to remember which foot goes first when you go up or down the stairs is to think of the phrase: **'Up with the good, down with the bad.'** When you go UP stairs, you lead with your good leg, so place your non-injured leg on the next step first. When you go DOWN stairs, you lead with your injured leg, so you place your injured leg on the next step first.

Stairs without a handrail

If the stairs have no handrail you're effectively walking as you normally would, but you're going up or down steps in the process. Once again, it may be helpful to follow these simple reminders:

- The crutches stay with the injured leg.

- Up with the good.

- Down with the bad.

So to go up a step, you **place your weight on your crutches through your arm and lift your good leg high enough to reach the next step**. Once your good leg is on the step, you put all your weight on it and follow with the crutches and the injured leg.

When you go down the stairs, you go down with the bad leg first, so the injured leg and the crutches are placed on the step first and then you follow with your good leg.

I realise this probably sounds a bit more complicated than it needs to be when written down, so it may be helpful to watch the video 'Non Weight Bearing on Stairs using Crutches' by Kaiser Permanente Santa Rosa on YouTube if you're at all unsure. **Whenever possible, always be sure to ask your physiotherapist or healthcare professional to show you what to do when you first start using crutches**.

Bathing and showering

Showering with a non-weight-bearing leg when you're using crutches is another tricky task, especially at first. Don't forget that if you've been lying down for a few days like I was – either waiting for the surgery or recovering from it – you may also be feeling a little weak. You could be feeling dizzy when you get up, as your blood pressure might be considerably lower than usual, so be careful when you get in the shower. Ensure you've been standing for a bit and don't feel dizzy or lightheaded before stepping in. Plus, you're probably still getting used to your crutches, and if your shower has a step you might find this a little tricky too.

If you need to have a bath in the first few days, you may find it helpful to get yourself to the side of it, turn your back towards it as you would when sitting on a chair and then sit on the side. Once you've positioned your crutches somewhere within reach, you can slide both your legs into the bath, and use your good foot and your arms to lower the rest of your body inside. **Be very careful not to slip during this process.** If at all possible, consider asking your partner or a relative for help. To get out, you reverse the process. Use your good foot and arms to pull yourself to the side, sit down and get both your legs out of the bath.

When getting in and out of the shower or bath, remember that:

- You want to leave your crutches in a place where they won't get wet (for example, just outside the shower). However, they need to be somewhere where you can easily reach them when you come out again. This is most definitely a no-hopping situation!

- You want to have a towel close by so that you can dry your hands and arms before you use your crutches. Wet hands and crutches really don't mix well.

- You need to be extra careful of wet and slippery surfaces. Crutches slip on wet floors and mats. Be careful of where you put them – you always need to ensure the crutches have a good grip on the floor.

See section 9 for other accessories that might help you with washing (including a shower chair and a waterproof leg cover).

Carrying things

Being on crutches unfortunately means that you can't really use your hands for anything else when you're walking. Depending on your lifestyle and living conditions, you may see this as a big obstacle at first. If you live on your own, you can't even carry a hot cup of coffee from the kitchen over to the sofa! Hopping with a hot drink in your hands is certainly not the solution! So how do you carry things around the house?

- **Get a backpack**. While this doesn't work for the aforementioned coffee or a plate of food, it will work for most other things. If you need to get changed after your shower, for example, pack all your stuff and take it to the bathroom with you. Another option is to use a small cross body bag, but if you do, make sure it doesn't interfere with your crutches.

- **Keep a box or bucket** by the side of your bed or sofa. This is where you want to keep things like the remote control, your phone charger, medication or anything that you may need when you're sitting down with your leg propped up. Just have all these little things by your side so you can easily grab them when you need them.

- **Use any surfaces available to you.** This one is probably a bit tricky to explain, but say I had to get something from the fridge and bring it over to the kitchen counter, I'd let go of one crutch (leaving it hanging from my arm by the cuff), standing by the fridge, get my item and with the help of my good leg and one crutch I'd move my good foot side to side to walk towards the counter. Then I'd lean on the counter with one hand, move a step, grab the item, put it further down onto the counter, lean on the counter again and keep going that way. The key is that I wouldn't hop (not with the milk carton in my hand anyway!) Does it take forever? Yes. It is a pain to have to do this? Totally. Does it work? Yes, it gets the job done eventually. Is it safe? Yes. And that's always the main thing at this stage of your recovery.

Over time, and when you feel confident enough, you'll be able to grab something light and not too bulky between your thumb and your index finger, while still using your crutches, and take it with you. This could be a light plastic bag, a snack bar or an item of clothing, for example. But be careful when doing this, as even when something seems easy to carry, it can throw you off balance when you use crutches. And you most definitely don't want to lose the grip on your crutch handle, or you'll end up falling flat on your face. So at first just hold on to those hand grips for dear life and forget about carrying anything.

Other safety considerations

As you've probably realised by now, crutches do take some getting used to! It will be tricky to move around the house at first, let alone navigate steps and stairs and venturing outdoors. Aside from the risk of injuring your arms and wrists, crutches put you at an increased risk of slipping. To prevent this from happening you can take the following precautions:

- Try to remove clutter and keep floors clean and dry – you may need some assistance with all this, so have a think about how this could be done for you. When people call and ask how they can help, this is something they can definitely do for you!

- Make sure any mats and rugs are secured onto the ground so you don't trip over them. They can be slippery, so do consider temporarily removing them if you can.

- Remember not to walk on wet or slippery surfaces – before you take a step, always make sure the rubber tips at the bottom of your crutches have a good grip on the floor.

They are meant to be non-slip, but they don't mix well with water.

- When you walk, try to look ahead rather than at your feet. This helps you with not losing your balance. At the same time though, you've got to watch where you're going. The last thing you want is to put your crutch somewhere where it can get stuck, like on a treacherous or uneven surface for example, or somewhere that doesn't give you a good grip.

- It will be tempting to hop around on your good leg, especially if you're just going, say, from the sink to the fridge. **Do not hop!** You can slip, lose your balance (and end up putting weight on your injured leg to avoid falling) or risk hurting your good leg or arms. I know of people who fell over when hopping. You just don't need this right now.

- When you're not using your crutches, rest them on the floor next to you if you can. Be sure to leave them where it's easy for you to reach them again. Remember it's best not to hop anywhere without your crutches!

- Go barefoot or use non-slip socks on your good foot around the house, and avoid using slippers, sandals or flip flops that might fall off. Shop around for good-quality socks with a good grip – they will make all the difference, especially if you have wooden or tiled flooring at home.

- Walking on crutches puts your upper body under additional stress. Be mindful of trying to keep your shoulders back and down to avoid upper back and neck pain.

- If you have any steps around the house, follow the same instructions as for managing stairs. Take your time, and remember that staying safe and injury-free is now your main concern. As you get more and more confident on crutches, navigating steps and stairs will become second nature to you.

Accessories for your crutches

There are all sorts of accessories you can get for your crutches. Just head over to Amazon and take your pick. You'll find:

- Crutch pods. These are little containers that you can attach to your crutches to carry small objects in.

- Padded handle covers.

- Crutch belts to hold your crutches over your shoulders while you're standing still and leaning against a surface, for example.

- Crutch holders, to keep your crutches together and hang them somewhere when you're not using them.

Do you absolutely need any of these things? Probably not. I didn't, but I did look into them to see if I could find anything to make my life easier. If you find something that you think can help and you can afford it, then go for it!

With the pods, be mindful of the fact you're adding weight to your crutches, and that could affect your balance. If you like to walk around outdoors to improve your confidence with your crutches or just to break up the monotony of being stuck at home, a padded handle cover might be a good idea for you. Without one, it's likely that the skin on your hands might become toughened or sore as a result of repeated friction and pressure of your hands on the crutch handles. This is normal to an extent, but if it bothers you the protectors might be a solution.

As for crutch belts or holders, well – crutches fall *all the time*. They are an absolute pain – either you put them directly on the floor, or if you rest them against any surface you can be sure at least one of them will fall over! Personally, after a lot of research I decided against any of the accessories so I can't recommend them based on my own experience, but it's worth having a look to see what's available and whether they can help you in any way.

8. Your follow-up appointments

Depending on where you are in the world, your age and your individual circumstances, you'll probably be given your first follow-up appointment a few weeks after surgery. Mine was six weeks after the operation, but it could be different for you.

At this appointment you may be offered X-rays as this is the best way for your doctor to check how your bone is healing. All being well you won't be in as much pain as you were when you first broke your leg, so you shouldn't worry too much about this appointment. You'll be able to move your leg much better on the table this time. But don't be too surprised (or too hard on yourself) if being in the room brings back some bad memories!

Your doctor may also perform what they refer to as a 'clinical check,' i.e. a combination of observations and 'manipulations.' So they'll observe how you handle yourself and move your leg, for example, and might ask for your permission to manipulate your leg. At my six-week check, the orthopaedist pressed quite hard on my leg with both hands. I must admit I was a bit apprehensive, but to my surprise it wasn't painful. Judging from the progress he could see on the X-rays and these clinical observations, he concluded I was making good progress and my fracture was healing as expected.

Up until this point I had been non-weight-bearing, so when he asked me to put partial weight on my leg, I found the exercise quite difficult. At the end of this appointment, I was told I could put partial pressure (between 30–50% of my weight) on the injured leg.

No matter at what stage of your recovery you are, **remember to ask questions at your follow-up appointments**. They are the only chance you have to see a specialist, so **make sure you write all your questions down in advance and bring them with you to your appointment**. You may think you don't need to do this and that you'll remember all the questions you want to ask, but trust me – it's very easy for your mind to go blank at your appointment.

For example, you may want to ask the specialist:

- How much weight you can put on your leg, and how you judge how much is too much.

- Why are you experiencing any particular symptoms? (Write them down in advance and remember to ask!) For example, you could ask about pain or discomfort in certain areas, numbness, dry skin, discoloration, etc.

- Can you exercise? Swim? Use gym equipment?

The number and frequency of your checks may vary according to where you are and your own personal situation. To give you an idea, my follow-up appointments (in the UK) were at:

- Six weeks – I went from non-weight-bearing to partial weight-bearing.

- 14 weeks – I went from partial weight-bearing to full weight-bearing.

- 20 weeks – I was discharged from the orthopaedic department at the hospital and started driving a week later.

9. Accessories and home adaptations

Adjustable toilet frame

You probably never even noticed this before in your life, but now you're injured you'll find out that toilets are generally quite low. Lowering yourself to sit down on the toilet with a non-weight-bearing leg and crutches might feel quite difficult at first.

An adjustable toilet frame or 'surround rail' could help you with this problem. If you are in the UK, get in touch with the Occupational Therapy team at your hospital. They provide support to people with health conditions that prevent them from doing everyday activities. If you're not in the UK, ask your doctor – there might be a team with a similar remit where you live. In the UK, Occupational Therapy may be able to lend you some of the equipment you need for free. Otherwise, it might be possible for you to hire or buy a specific item. Whichever option you choose, be sure to check the toilet frame's measurements first. They tend to be quite large, so you want to make sure you have enough space around the toilet to comfortably position one.

With a frame, when you need to use the toilet you can lean on it and use your arms and upper body strength to safely lower yourself onto the seat. To get up, simply reverse the process. You grab the frame, push yourself up, make sure you have your balance first, then grab your crutches and off you go.

Raised toilet seat

A raised (and padded) toilet seat will also help you when you're trying to sit on the toilet by making it higher. Once again, you may be able to borrow this for free from your hospital (speak to Occupational Therapy or equivalent) – you'll return all equipment when you no longer need it. Otherwise, you may be able to hire or buy one. Like the toilet frame, it isn't a must-have but everything that can make your life a little easier for those first weeks while you're non-weight-bearing is in my opinion worthwhile.

Shower chair or stool

Balancing on one leg when you're having a shower can be a bit tiring. Plus, you don't want to risk losing your balance or slipping while you're washing your hair. A shower chair or stool could come in very handy for the first few weeks. Once again, my amazing Occupational Therapy team at the hospital provided me with one I could use for free until I was better, but you can consider hiring or buying one.

Waterproof leg or cast cover

If you have a cast or dressing, you'll definitely need a waterproof leg cover to make sure it doesn't get wet when you have a shower. You can make do with any large plastic bag, making sure that you tie it tightly at the top so that your leg cannot get wet. This may be a bit difficult to do though, so you could invest in a waterproof cast and dressing protector.

Putting it on can be tricky at first. As the biggest incision for my surgery was on my knee it was hard to bend it enough to be able to reach my foot and put the cover on. If you have someone at home with you, ask them to help. However, in the end I found that doing it myself was better simply because I knew where and when I felt pain, and I could regulate my actions accordingly. It wasn't the most pleasant of tasks, but you have to remember that you'll only need the cover while you have your dressing on (or while you have a cast), so it'll only be for a few weeks. Once you're finished using the leg cover, I'd suggest hanging it somewhere upside down to dry, ready for the next use.

Adjustable chair with armrest

An adjustable chair is a seat (without wheels) whose height you can adjust. It has armrests, so you can lean on it to sit yourself down or get up again. It may come in handy at the dinner table, the kitchen counter or the sink if you find standing and balancing on one leg too tiring and prefer to sit down. It may be of help in those first few weeks, and you can hire or buy one.

10. Helping the healing process

Although your tibia (and fibula, if it was fractured) will still take a number of weeks to fully heal, your health, wellbeing, diet and lifestyle will have a considerable impact on how quickly and successfully you recover. What you do during this time has the potential to influence how quickly, comfortably and well your bones heal.

I will summarise the key points from my research in the following sections, but if you want to read some excellent and detailed information on bone health and the healing process, I thoroughly recommend the website betterbones.com by Dr Susan E. Brown, and in particular the article 'How to speed fracture healing.' Another website I'd encourage you to visit when it comes to learning about diet and nutrition is draxe.com by Dr Josh Axe.

10.1 Your diet

Before we get into the details here, it's important to note that while the advice below is designed to help you during the recovery process, the following dietary and lifestyle changes will actually help you strengthen your entire skeleton and improve your overall health. In other words, it wouldn't hurt you to continue to follow this advice even after you've fully recovered from your fracture and 'gone back to normal.' After all, if your particular circumstances call for the tibial IM nail to be removed at a later date (more on that in section 13), you want your bones to be at their strongest and healthiest!

As you'll see, ideally you want your diet to include a lot of vegetables, fruit and some organic meat, as well as nuts and seeds.

Increasing your caloric intake

Fracture healing is hard work for your body! You may think that because you're not moving around much your body isn't consuming a lot of energy right now, but the opposite is true. While your broken bones are being repaired, you consume additional calories. An active adult may require approximately 2,500 calories per day, but during your recovery you should aim to increase your caloric intake to 6,000 or thereabouts. In other words, you need to eat!

Increasing your protein intake

When we look at skeletal composition, roughly half of bone is made of protein. When a fracture occurs, in very simplistic terms the body needs protein (and minerals) to rebuild that bone. If you starve your body of one of the key building blocks required to knit your bones back together, you may inadvertently delay your recovery or, worse, even experience complications. In other words, getting enough protein ensures your body has what it needs to repair and restore itself.

One of the key types of protein you're going to need is **collagen**. This contributes to the mechanical strength of our bones. It helps to build bone matrix, repair connective tissues for improved elasticity, improve blood circulation and promote wound healing. Foods that contain collagen are fish, red, dark green and orange vegetables and berries, for example. If you wish, consider speaking to your doctor about introducing a supplement.

Increasing anti-inflammatory nutrients

Inflammation, although painful, is the first stage of bone healing. It's the body's own method for repairing damage. What's important in this phase are nutrients that are anti-inflammatory and nourishing to new bone growth. Useful anti-inflammatory nutrients are antioxidants, including vitamin E and vitamin C and omega-3 fatty acids (for this, consider fish oil supplements). These nutrients naturally help soothe the inflammatory process and speed up healing. They are needed because the trauma of the fracture itself causes 'oxidative stress' that can negatively impact the body's antioxidant reserves.

Increasing your mineral intake

Together with protein, minerals are the building blocks for bone re-building. As most of us probably don't consume enough minerals on an everyday basis, following a healthy diet that pays particular attention to our mineral intake during the recovery process couldn't be more important.

The key minerals involved in the process are:

- **Zinc** – enhances bone protein production and stimulates fracture healing. Zinc-rich dishes are similar to calcium- and magnesium-rich foods and include grass-fed beef, pumpkin seeds, chia and flaxseeds.

- **Copper** – aids in the formation of bone collagen.

- **Calcium and phosphorus** – fundamental to the building and rebuilding of bone tissue. A calcium deficiency can actually contribute to broken bones! In order to start healing your fractures, your body draws on its available reserves, but to not deplete them, you need to ensure you consume plenty of calcium-rich foods in your diet. Calcium absorption is dependent on vitamin D, so this is another important nutrient for you right now. You can get calcium from green leafy foods such as spinach, broccoli and kale.

- **Magnesium** – because calcium and magnesium work in very close conjunction with each other, in order for your body to use calcium you have to have magnesium. You can find it in green leafy vegetables, flaxseeds, chia seeds and pumpkin seeds, for example, as well as almonds, avocados and black beans.

- **Silicon** – this is found in fruit, whole grains (especially bran and oats) and vegetables such as carrots, spinach, beetroot and string beans. It helps with the formation of collagen, the tough fibrous material that play an essential role in bone health and regeneration, as well as supporting healthy skin and strong hair.

If in doubt, speak to your doctor about introducing supplements to your diet to ensure you fuel your body with plenty of these nutrients.

Increasing vitamin intake

These vitamins have been identified as playing a key role in the fracture healing process:

- **Vitamin C** plays a fundamental part in bone collagen formation and is required for fracture healing. Think oranges, lemons, bell peppers, kiwis, broccoli, asparagus, vegetable juices and orange juice.

- **Vitamin D** is the primary regulator of calcium absorption, and without adequate vitamin D calcium blood levels drop, making less calcium available for fracture healing. In other words, a vitamin D deficiency can hinder the healing of your broken bone(s). So if you can't get yourself out in the sunshine, consider talking to your doctor about taking a daily supplement.

- **Vitamin K** helps conserve calcium by reducing the loss of it in the urine.

- **Vitamin B6** is one of the B vitamins that has been linked to fracture healing.

Lysine

When reading up about the healing process, I found that a specific amino acid called lysine is known to enhance calcium absorption, increase the amount of calcium absorbed into the bone matrix and aid in the regeneration of tissue. After checking with my doctor, they confirmed that they couldn't see any reason why I shouldn't take a supplement, so I did. Before doing so, be sure to check with your doctor that these are safe and appropriate for you.

Smoking

Smoking is detrimental to the bone repair process because it reduces blood circulation. According to information from betterbones.com, patients who smoke take longer to heal than patients who don't. Smoking also increases the incidence of the risks associated with the intramedullary nail surgery, including delayed healing, infection and non-union.

Alcohol

In order to give yourself the best chances to recover as quickly as possible, it's also advisable to reduce the amount of alcohol you consume, if any. Similarly to smoking, drinking excessive amounts of alcohol can increase the risk of developing complications associated with your surgery, including delayed healing and infection.

Other foods to avoid

During your recovery, it's particularly important to stay away from foods that tend to be overly acidic (including non-organic meat and dairy products) as well as from excess salt and sugar. These will acidify your body, leach minerals out of your system and cause your bone healing and growth to slow down.

Alternative and natural healing aids

Before modern medicine made the resources and medications we have today, the traditional methods for healing broken bones were based on **herbs and plants**. Different types of complementary and alternative medicine (also known as CAM) may now come into their own. So, if you're willing to look into further resources that may add to the medical care you're receiving, here are some practices you may want to find out more about:

- Chinese medicine, including acupuncture. This helps re-direct where your body energy is being utilised, thus supporting repair to damaged bones.

- Herbal medicine.

- Ayurvedic medicine.

- Homeopathic remedies.

If you do decide to explore these avenues in the context of bone healing and strengthening, ensure you **follow the guidance and advice of qualified practitioners in these areas** (herbalists, homeopaths, etc.) and **always consult your doctor** to discuss any potential risks or side effects that you may need to be aware of.

In terms of specific herbs and plants that *may* help, some of the alternative remedies worth looking into are:

- Arnica (*arnica montana*) – it helps after a trauma with pain and swelling.

- Symphytum (comfrey) for pain relief and bone repair.

- Horsetail grass is a herb high in silicon, which can be boiled and made into a tea. It's said to be valuable especially in the early stages of fracture healing.

- Cissus quadrangularis is an Indian herb that's been studied for its fracture-healing benefits.

- Turmeric – helps support a healthy inflammatory response as well as heart, joint and liver functions. You can add turmeric spices to foods, take a supplement to promote healing or just buy the root, peel it, grate it and add it to hot water or tea.

- Apple cider vinegar is considered to be a strong remedy for illnesses and a precious tool to increase overall health. Consider taking it daily mixed in warm water.

- Zheng Gu Shui. This is a brand of traditional Chinese pain relief liniment used to treat bone fractures and breaks – literally translated, the name means 'fix bone water' or 'rectify bone water.' Fitness coach Caroline Jordan from carolinejordanfitness.com describes this as a "liniment especially designed to relieve pain associated with fractures, bruises and other types of mild trauma. I put the ointment on my foot nightly and also found it helpful with sore muscles, aches and pains."

During your recovery, you may also want to investigate these non-conventional energy healing methods: **reiki, qi gong, polarity therapy, healing touch, acupuncture, and massage**. I have no personal experience of these, but they are worth a try if you believe that any of these practices may help.

When your wounds have healed enough so that you can get your leg wet, consider taking regular Epsom salt baths. This is naturally high in magnesium and sulphates, and when these minerals are absorbed into the skin they can help you deal with pain, relax your muscles and promote blood circulation and recovery. Epsom salt also helps to flush toxins, improve absorption of nutrients and form joint proteins.

Another option to look into are essential oils with anti-inflammatory powers. According to Dr Axe from draxe.com, the following oils should help your fractured bones heal faster:

- Cypress – helps to improve circulation in the area.

103

- Fir needle – helps to repair the bone.

- Helychrisum – has anti-inflammatory and antioxidant properties, so it helps to repair damaged nerve tissue due.

As long as you have no wounds around the fractured area caused by the injury, you can make a blend with these oils and apply it to your skin five or six times a day. However, only do this under the advice and guidance of an essential oils advocate in your area. The company dōTERRA at doterra.com may be a good place to start. However, do make sure you **never apply essential oils on broken or wounded skin (including your surgery incisions)**.

10.2 Rest, exercise, and maintaining a healthy mind

The best thing you can do in the first few days and couple of weeks after your accident is to **follow your body's cues and rest when you need to**. You're using up a lot of energy to fix your broken bones right now. Plus, you may also still feel drowsy or weak as a result of the surgery and the medications you've been taking, and to top all that off you're also putting a lot of additional strain on your upper body while mastering the art of walking on crutches. **Go easy on yourself!** Nothing is gained in the long run by exhausting yourself now and doing too much too soon. The last thing you need at this point is to get hurt or fall ill.

If your situation at home allows it, take the time to literally put your feet up (remember that it's good for helping with blood circulation and preventing swelling?) and read a book or watch some TV. Now is the time to rest, relax and give yourself a break (excuse the pun). This will pay dividends later. In a few weeks, things will look a lot easier. You'll be stronger and more mobile. It's hard, but you just need to be a little patient until then.

Exercise

Exercise is unlikely to pop into your mind as an important way to accelerate fracture healing, but it is. Fracture healing requires **good circulation and an adequate flow of nutrient-replenishing blood to the fracture site**, both of which are enhanced by exercise. Of course you should only follow exercises that have been recommended to you by your physiotherapist or a qualified instructor who fully understands your condition.

It goes without saying that if you choose to exercise, you should avoid putting excessive weight on your injured leg too soon and keep yourself safe. If you bear this in mind, exercising will:

- Help you maintain mobility in your ankle and knee.

- Minimise pain and swelling in your joints.

- Help you maintain your weight while you're not able to walk or exercise as usual.

- Increase your bone density (through weights).

- Help you with your mental wellbeing.

Physiotherapy

Depending on where you live, your hospital may recommend you attend regular physiotherapy appointments to help you **maintain or regain muscle strength, movement and flexibility**. How soon after your surgery you will start physiotherapy sessions will largely depend on the local protocol of where you live and on your age, health, and level of fitness. Whenever you start to work with a physiotherapist, you'll be given specific exercises that will be appropriate to your specific situation and stage of recovery.

It's important you don't try to rush your recovery by returning to your normal activities too quickly, as your broken bone may not be fully healed even when the pain has gone. Always be sure to follow your doctor or physiotherapist's advice, who'll probably recommend **gradually increasing how much you can use your leg over time**.

While you're non-weight-bearing for the first four to six weeks at least, and if you're not wearing a cast, you'll be able to do some very simple exercises that will help you maintain a good range of motion and not lose mobility in your knee and your ankle, provided that there is nothing wrong with them. The last thing you want is for your knee and ankle to become stiff and lose the ability to move, as this will be a lot harder (and painful) to reverse later on. The fitter you stay now, and the more you try to maintain mobility and muscle strength, the quicker you'll literally be back on your feet when you're ready to bear weight on your leg again.

So if you can (i.e. your injury allows it, and you don't have a cast), consider doing the following:

- Ankle pumps.

- Rotating your ankle(s).

- Bending your toes – together and independently.

- Bending your knee.

- Calf stretches – as long as and as soon as these feel comfortable.

There is a fair chance you'll be told you can swim – this is probably the best form of exercise for you right now, and one of the only ones you can do without bearing weight on your leg. However, remember you need to be able to get yourself by the pool and in and out of the water safely. When on crutches (and walking on wet, slippery floors) consider getting some help.

If you feel well enough, a few weeks after your surgery you can start to exercise your upper body as long as you're always careful to put the right amount of weight on your injured leg, or no amount of weight at all if you're still non-weight-bearing. Have a look on YouTube for 'non-weight-bearing leg exercises' or 'non-weight-bearing workout' and you'll find several videos for inspiration. Remember though – always check with a professional and ensure any exercises or movements are appropriate for your circumstances.

In cases of delayed union (i.e. when the segments of the bone are not knitting together as quickly or as well as they could), rehabilitation may also include vibration therapy. While the patient stands on a special platform, mechanical vibration (i.e. energy) is sent through the body. The vibrations help muscles to contract and blood circulation to increase. Vibration platforms can be used for some patients to promote healing. Check with your physiotherapist or doctor to see whether this could be a viable option for you.

Your mental health, attitude, and mindset

- Be kind to yourself. Tuning into your body and responding to your energy levels will help you with your emotional and mental health too. In the first couple of weeks, you may have bad days – the pain and discomfort may prevent you from resting well at night, and you might often feel frustrated at your situation. Try to accept that some days may feel a little harder, and be compassionate to yourself. Try to steer away from focusing on the 'what if' – it will just bring up and fuel negative thoughts, feelings and emotions, and right now this is quite blatantly a waste of your energy.

- Lower your expectations. You need to start coming to terms with the fact that in the very first days and weeks of your recovery, especially while you're non-weight-bearing, you won't be able to do things the way you've always done them. This can be hard when you're used to being the one looking after other people, for example, but think about stripping your life back to the basics, and before you do something ask yourself whether it *absolutely* needs to be done *right now* and *by you*. If not, leave it. It may be hard for you to do right now, but remember that it's only temporary.

- Stay positive. There's a very strong connection between your mind and body. The more you can stay positive, patient and focused on what you can do to help yourself and make progress, the better your recovery will feel. Do whatever works for you to lift your spirits and take positive steps towards recovery. As hard as it can be some days, trust the journey and your body. It's not always easy to grasp how you're going to cope in this situation for five or six months, but things do improve! So if it helps, try not to look at the end goal for now. Focus on the next milestone instead. If you have a doctor's visit coming up in three weeks, for example, focus on that. Keep your mind focused on whatever *you* can do to help your body do its job and heal.

- Try to embrace it. Think about how you can use this time. What happened to you isn't a good thing by any stretch of the imagination, but unfortunately it has happened. So how can you use this opportunity?

  - Can you learn anything from this experience and start doing something differently?

  - Does this make you look at your life or yourself in a different light?

  - How can you use this time?

  - What dietary and lifestyle changes can you make that will help you become healthier in the long run?

Personally, I've never been one to exercise much, but during my six-week check my specialist said I could start to bear partial weight on my injured leg, and it was safe for me to use my exercise bike at home, *as long as I didn't feel any pain in my injured leg*, so I started to use the exercise bike daily. It helped me keep my weight under control and strengthen my leg muscles, as well as encouraging good mobility in the knee of my injured leg. Doing something practical towards my healing and recovery was the incentive I needed to finally start using the exercise bike! It gave me a purpose, a positive challenge and the sense I was doing something good and useful for myself. I was no longer a 'victim of the situation' – I was taking responsibility, taking charge of my own health, and this massively helped with my emotional and mental wellbeing.

Although it may not seem like that right now, this could be an opportunity for you to grow stronger and more resilient both mentally and physically.

- Ask for and accept help. Yes, you'll have to eventually learn to do things by yourself, but if you can, especially at first, ask for and accept any help you may be offered. Remember, you don't want to be a hero and hurt yourself even further. Things will get a lot easier when you can put partial weight on your injured leg.

- Try to surround yourself with positive, supportive people. Your injury may mean you're now spending extra time alone, and that isn't always helpful. If you can, invite people over or take the opportunity to get in touch with old friends you haven't spoken to in ages. If it helps, go online and see if you can find someone in a similar situation – each case is different, but it may help to 'compare notes' and have someone to talk to who understands what you're going through. An easy way to do this is to go on Twitter and do a search with the hashtags #brokenleg, #brokentibia or #brokenfibula (if you broke your fibula too). At the time of writing, a Facebook group called 'Intramedullary Nail/IM Nail/Tibia Nail/Rod' exists. If you request to join, you can interact with others who are or have been in a similar situation.

- **Get out of the house.** If you can, try to **spend some time outdoors in nature**. Do this regularly, if possible. Of course, no one is suggesting you go hiking or trekking at this stage of your recovery, but try to spend some time in the garden, a local park or anywhere you can be surrounded by trees, if you can do so safely. Huge benefits come from being outdoors in nature, including:

  - A boosted immune system (don't you just need that right now?)

  - Improved mood and reduced stress.

  - Accelerated recovery from surgery or illness.

  - Increased energy levels.

  - Improved sleep.

  - Increased flow of energy and sense of happiness.

The last thing you need right now is to experience 'cabin fever' and feel irritable and restless because you're stuck indoors, so get out and have some fun!

11. Going from non-weight-bearing to partial weight-bearing

Congratulations! You've reached a massive milestone in your recovery. How long after surgery this happens may be different for everyone, but at this point in your recovery your specialist will advise you that your leg is now strong enough for you to be able to put **partial weight** on it. You may now start to walk with one crutch only, at least some of the time. This is great news, but if you started off as non-weight-bearing or light-touch weight-bearing, partial weight-bearing will take some caution and getting used to at first. Once you get a feel for how much weight you can put on your leg though, using one crutch instead of two will give you one arm and a hand back and you'll really see a big difference in your day-to-day mobility.

By now (and if you started off with two crutches) you're probably used to crutches anyway and life will start to feel a lot easier. You also probably know how to handle yourself and your crutches a lot better than you used to. You're no longer in the same place you were when you first got home from hospital after surgery!

How much weight is 'partial weight'?

To give you an idea, when I was advised that I could start bearing partial weight on my injured leg (six weeks post-op), I was told I could apply between 20% and 50% of my weight on my injured leg. After spending six weeks being light-touch weight-bearing, it was hard for me to judge how much weight I could put on my leg at first, but over time you get a feel for it.

When you reach this milestone, **be sure to ask your doctor to clarify how much weight you can put on your leg**. If they give you a percentage like they gave me, be prepared to have to experiment a little before you feel confident you're doing the right thing.

The advice the orthopaedist gave me was to be guided by the pain I experienced – pain equals too much weight too soon. If you are in doubt as to what you should do, make sure you speak to your doctor or physiotherapist and take their advice. Your tibia is healing – you're getting quite far along into your recovery, and you don't want to do anything to compromise this.

Walking on one crutch

The correct way to walk with one crutch is to:

- **Place the crutch on the arm opposite your injured leg**. So if you hurt your right leg, for example, you should use your one crutch with your left arm. If you hurt your left leg, use your crutch with your right arm.

- **Move the crutch forward and step with your injured leg at the same time** – part of your weight will fall on your injured leg, and the other part will be supported by your upper body and crutch.

- **Keep the crutch close to your body** for support and balance.

When you're able to put more weight on your leg (i.e. you become partial weight-bearing or can put full weight on your injured leg again), you may still need physiotherapy. Your foot, ankle, and muscles will be weak from the lack of walking over the last few weeks or months. It's important that you regularly carry out the exercises outlined by your physiotherapist to be able to get back to full strength. These will include stretches and simple balancing exercises designed to strengthen the specific muscles that were weakened during your recovery.

If you've been discharged by a specialist after your tibia has fully healed, but you feel you've not regained full mobility, are still experiencing pain or discomfort or limping, make sure you speak to your doctor and ask for support. A few months may have now passed from your injury, but it's important you keep working on strengthening your leg until it feels good again.

12. 'Back to normal'

Massive congratulations! You've now reached THE milestone of going from partial weight-bearing to full weight-bearing! You've done it! It's over! You're now 'back to normal.' Or are you?

You've just been to your last appointment, and your surgeon just told you that your bones have successfully healed and you can now ditch the crutches and literally walk out of the hospital on your own two feet. It should feel amazing. It IS amazing! But you have **mixed feelings**. You're happy, of course. This is fantastic news, and everything you'd be waiting to hear for weeks (months, even), but somehow your leg doesn't feel 'normal' yet. Sure, it's no longer your *broken leg*, but it's not the same as your other leg either and it certainly isn't the same it was before. Not yet anyway.

In addition, you might not be feeling quite your old self either. Physically, you may have put on a little weight (after being forced to lead a more sedentary lifestyle), and emotionally you may also be experiencing a small degree of **anxiety** over returning to work or going back to doing things you haven't done in a while, such as driving, playing sports or engaging in physical activities. You may even be worried about going back to doing whatever it was you did when you got injured.

If you feel vulnerable, anxious or unsure as to what you can or can't do when you start to bear full weight on your injured leg again, you should know you're not alone. Like most of us, you probably expected 'getting back to normal' to be a lot better than this. You expected your leg to feel and function much better than it is right now. But don't worry, you'll get there. It may just take a little longer. This 'normal' you're now experiencing will change and for the better.

To give you an idea of what I mean by this, I'll give you some examples of how my leg didn't feel very 'normal' after I had been told my tibia had fully healed at my 20 week post-op appointment:

- I had a visible limp that I only managed to address with the help and care of a physiotherapist. The limp stayed with me until about six months after my injury and was caused by the weakening, shortening and tightening of my foot and leg muscles due to inactivity and lack of walking.

- I had pain in the sole of my foot and my toes, and my foot and ankle would often swell up as a result of walking. Again, this was due to weakened foot muscles because of the lack of walking over the past few months.

- Probably due to temporary nerve damage caused by the surgery, I found that I couldn't bend my big toe, but after about six months the issue resolved itself. This obviously affected the way I walked at the time.

- I experienced considerable pain at the back of my leg (my calf muscles) when walking. Again, this was due to muscle weakness and shortening caused by the lack of activity, but it really did affect the way I was walking (and limping).

- With all the above issues, I was also unable to run (or even jog) until six to seven months after the surgery, and it took me a while longer to even feel confident enough to try.

- I was completely unable to stand on my tiptoes/forefoot, balancing on my injured leg until about seven or eight months after surgery.

- If I stand on the leg or walk for long periods of time it swells up, especially at the ankle, and starts to feel really uncomfortable to the point where I may limp the following day. The same happens on long-haul flights.

- The scars from the surgery still felt quite sensitive, especially the one on my knee (it still does, 16 months after surgery, although it's a lot better), and I can't kneel on the floor. I'm told this one is there to stay.

- An area about 5cm (2in) wide at the side of my leg has no sensitivity. This may have been due to nerve damage that could have occurred during surgery. I was informed that sensation may or may not return. If it does, it may take years for it to do so.

- My leg is *very* sensitive to cold and wet weather, and on those days it feels stiff, slightly sore and just somehow 'not right.'

- When I drive for over 45 minutes or so or if I run, I become quite aware of the screws in my ankle. I feel a dull burning sensation in that area.

Over time and with simple stretches recommended by the physiotherapists, some of these symptoms have improved. While I can certainly say that my life is 'back to normal' (after all, I can do all the everyday things I was doing before my accident), I feel very apprehensive about my leg. I am very aware of having a big piece of titanium in it, and although I go about my normal life, I do feel a degree of minor anxiety around my limb. When I'm in a crowd or very close to other people I worry that someone will bump into my knee, for example. And although I know other people with a nail who do, I wouldn't dream of taking part in certain sports or physical activities in case I fall and hurt myself.

You may or may not relate to this, as how you feel will largely depend on your personality, your lifestyle, how you injured yourself and even what you do for a living. If you're a professional athlete and you injured yourself 'on the job,' you may just want to get back to it and do things I'd never even attempt in my dreams! But if you do experience these feelings and think this isn't how you used to be, it may reassure you to know that you're not alone.

One of the things you may want to consider is whether you think you'd feel a lot better if you had the nail removed, if this a possibility for you – more on that in section 13.

(Mindful) walking

As soon as your leg is strong enough to bear weight you can start walking again. Don't be surprised if this isn't going to be an immediate, straightforward process. In a way, it's a bit like your body has 'forgotten' how to do it. Remember that for the last few months, you've not used certain muscles. You put weight onto other areas of your body, and instead you've had to make some major adjustments when it comes to a lot of everyday movements. When we normally walk, we don't consciously think about what we need to do to make the next step – your body knows what to do and when to do it. But after a few weeks of inactivity, you need to consciously re-train your body to walk again.

Some of your muscles or tendons will have been affected by the surgery and your inability to bear weight, which is why specific exercises will help. Something you can try in the meantime is 'mindful walking.' Make a point of going for a walk on your own, and do so outdoors if you can. Try to focus on your 'good' foot. How do you walk? What part of your foot touches the ground first? What pace do you set? Try to really focus on the sensations of your 'good' foot performing the act of walking, and then try to replicate it with your healing leg and foot.

If you can't, or if you're limping, try not to get frustrated. This is helping you highlight where in your healing leg you may be feeling pain, stiffness or discomfort. And if you can't adjust this by yourself, it's excellent feedback you can give to your physiotherapist. The better you're able to describe your symptoms, the more they can help you address your specific weaknesses to get you back to full health as quickly as possible. Write down your impressions after every walk while they're still fresh in your mind so that you have an accurate record to share with your physiotherapist.

Footwear

When you start walking again (i.e. you've been told your healing leg can now bear full weight), you should consider wearing 'sensible,' comfortable shoes, at least for a while. Ask your physiotherapist for advice or try 'barefoot' or 'minimalist' shoes. Typically, this type of footwear has a very thin sole, no arch support and little cushioning at the heel, so they don't force your feet into any sort of unnatural position or movement. Walking may be tricky at first, even without shoes. Your bones may have fully healed, but your muscles and tendons now need to get used to walking again. Plus you may be suffering from temporary nerve damage from the surgery, which impacts the way you walk. So be patient (yes, still), and try whatever type of shoe you feel works best for you right now.

Your doctor or physiotherapist may advise you to avoid heels for about six months. This is because while you're still getting used to walking, heels will force your muscles into more unnatural positions and the stretches caused by this type of footwear may cause you pain and discomfort. Of course you may not be in this situation, so just be guided by your body. If heels still hurt after eight months, do consider whether they are worth the pain.

Going back to work

If your circumstances allowed it, you may have returned to work when you were still on crutches. But if that wasn't possible, chances are you'll be going back when you're able to walk and drive again. This is another big milestone in your recovery, and another one that calls for a little patience and self-kindness. Whatever your routine was, you have probably been out of it for a few months and it'll take some getting used to at first. Even though months have passed, **you may find your leg still gets swollen and tired very easily, and you may need to elevate it at night or have a soothing bath.**

Now that you're walking again and so many months have passed since your surgery, people around you will assume you're fine – you are literally 'back on your feet.' Yet you might not feel fine or you're not the same person you were. Your leg still isn't behaving the way you'd want it to and other people don't see or understand that. They might not necessarily know that when you get home from work you have to prop your leg up and ice it to get rid of swelling and pain. It can be frustrating to have to explain this to others, as you won't be met with a lot of empathy anymore. They don't understand how you feel or what you're going through, so if you need to vent try to find some fellow patients (in person or online) – they'll happily listen to your predicaments, share their own stories and spare a word of encouragement. Failing that, you can email me directly at sara@mindyourmamma.com - I'm always happy to compare notes with others!

Going back to playing sports

How long after your injury you can go back to running or playing sports will largely depend on your lifestyle *before* you broke your leg. If you're an athlete or play a particular sport, you may need specific physiotherapy and rehabilitation to restore any strength you may have lost in your leg muscles. You may need to work with a professional personal trainer or coach to check for any overcompensation – as a result of your injury you may be putting more strain on your lower back or on your 'good' leg, knee and foot, for example. When you're back to full health you want to make sure the relevant tweaks are made so you can handle your body in the best way possible and without the risk of further injuries.

If you play contact sports, your doctor may advise you not to for a few more months. The hardware in your leg helped you heal better and quicker, but should you sustain another injury in the same leg, the nail could cause a lot of damage. If this is your case, you may be a good candidate for early hardware removal (see section 13 for more on this). As always, **be sure to follow your specialist's advice when it comes to resuming any type of physical activity.**

Bone strengthening

Even though your bones have now healed, you can continue to follow the lifestyle and dietary choices you've been making during your recovery (see section 10.1 on diet). Why? Because essentially you want your bones to stay healthy and grow stronger, especially if you're going to be facing more surgery at some point (potentially to remove the nail and screws, see section 13). So continue to **eat your greens, eat enough proteins (and avoid very low-calorie diets), get plenty of calcium, vitamin D, vitamin K, magnesium, zinc and omega-3 fats, maintain a healthy weight and consider taking a collagen supplement** if your doctor gives you the okay to do so.

While your diet plays a huge role, so does **exercise.** Ask your physiotherapist or a trained professional who understands your situation to show you safe **strength training and weight-bearing exercises you can do once your leg has fully healed.** The objective here is to help you build and maintain strong bones. Weight-bearing and high-impact exercises are important because they promote the formation of new bone. Increased bone mineral density and bone strength are good components for a healthy life when you're much older as they reduce the risk of osteoporosis and further fractures.

Your scars

By now your wounds will have probably healed to a satisfactory degree. New tissue will have started to grow and new skin will have begun to form over this tissue. You will have noticed the wounds getting smaller and scars forming. You may notice that the area itches, and after the scab has fallen off your skin looks stretched, discoloured or shiny.

The new skin that appears under your scab is less strong and flexible than your 'old skin.' Over time, if you had small incision-type scars where the screws were inserted, you may notice these will fade and even disappear. If they do, it could take as long as two years for this to happen. However, some scars never disappear completely. Even if you didn't have any wounds as a result of your injury (i.e. your fracture wasn't open), you'll have a rather long incision on your knee and this scar may take a lot longer to fade.

Once your scabs have fallen off naturally, and you can see you have no cuts or openings on your skin, you may want to apply petroleum jelly such as Vaseline or vitamin E-based creams or oils (such as Bio-Oil, for example) onto your skin to minimise scarring. However, if you're unsure speak to your doctor or nurse to confirm it is okay for you to do so. **You should never apply cream or oils to your open wounds.**

At first when the skin is still very new, try to avoid exposing the scars to direct sunlight. This is because your new skin cannot efficiently protect you from the effects of ultraviolet radiation, and it may burn easily. Plus, exposure to sunlight may cause permanent discolouration of your skin.

If you wish, once your wounds have completely healed and your scars don't show any openings, you may even want to look into applying essential oils onto your skin to reduce the appearance of your scars. Good candidates could be helychrisum, frankincense and lavender. Make sure you do some research as to which oils are best recommended for reducing scars and, crucially, how they should be applied to the skin.

13. Nail removal (hardware removal)

A question quite high up on the agenda for anyone with a nail, some screws and/or plates in their leg is whether the metalwork is there to stay or if it can come out at some point.

This question definitely cannot be answered by this book, as the answer will very much depend on your own personal circumstances and health. In addition to this, there isn't a lot of information available on this topic, but I will try to cover some of what we know, including some of the risks of the surgery.

- Hardware removal (HWR, i.e. the surgical removal of your intramedullary nail, interlocking screws and any plates) is NOT always possible. In some cases the hardware becomes embedded in the bone, and it just isn't viable to take it out without causing more damage. This is especially true if you needed plates to keep the bones together in the first place, or if a long time has passed and the bone has grown in such a way that it has embedded the metalwork.

- It may be possible to remove some of the hardware but not all of it, or to remove different pieces of hardware through different surgeries and at different times.

- An intramedullary nail CAN remain in place for life and never be surgically removed. However, there are also risks to keeping it in your body. Should another fall or injury occur, the bone would have lost its elasticity due to the piece of metal inside its marrow. This means it could shatter in such a way that it would be very difficult to repair.

- If you participate in contact sports (football, rugby or martial arts, etc.) and the chances of another similar injury are higher, your consultant *may*, in your case, recommend the earlier surgical removal of your hardware. However, the general advice for adults seems to be that **the nail should not be removed before 12 months from the date of the original surgery**. This is because if the tibia is too weak or hasn't fully healed, and the surgery is performed too soon after the original fracture, the tibia could break again during the extraction of the metalwork.

- Having said that, there's little understanding (from a patient perspective) of when the 'sweet spot' to take the nail out might be. While it's clear that taking it out too soon means the tibia isn't strong enough and might break again, waiting too long *could* make for a harder procedure as the metalwork may have become embedded within the bone, and taking it out could create further complications, if it is possible at all. You should ask your specialist for their advice and potentially consider getting second opinions.

- For patients who have been experiencing aches and pains (especially in the knee area), the extraction of the nail may not eradicate this problem. In other words, their pain may persist even after the metalwork has been removed.

- There is a risk that the nail could break while being extracted, in which case it would need to be left in place.

- Although the surgery to remove the metalwork is easier and more straightforward than the operation that put it in, it still carries risks, including the one associated with general anaesthetic and the possibility of developing an infection or blood clot.

You can read more about the available research on hardware removal and its effects on loptonline.com in the article 'Adult Lower Leg Fractures.'

Recovery after hardware removal surgery

Assuming that everything goes well with the removal of the metalwork, the recovery after this surgery is considerably easier and less taxing than the recovery following the original procedure. Some patients report no longer requiring painkillers and being able to put their full weight on their leg within a few days after surgery.

When personally discussing this with my consultant (although I haven't had my metalwork removed yet at the time of writing), I was advised that if I go for the hardware removal, I will probably need to use crutches for approximately six–eight weeks to protect the bone. This is because the removal of the interlocking screws effectively creates weakness in the bone, and you're more prone to injury and incurring another fracture. Having said that, patients who had this type of surgery report being able to walk without crutches (perhaps using an orthopaedic boot for support and protection) within a week or so. Some patients admitted to being able to drive a couple of weeks after the operation.

Part Three: Appendix

14. My story

I'm adding this section, as when I broke my leg I found it helpful to see what other people were experiencing — what they were going through and what worked for them. So here's my story.

The fall

I broke my right tibia and fibula on the 1 September 2016. I was carrying an empty suitcase down the stairs (wearing socks on carpet) and I slipped. I didn't roll down the stairs in a dramatic way, but basically I sat on my right leg with a bit of a forward motion — enough to twist the leg and crack the bones in the process.

I heard the crack, and as this wasn't my first fracture I immediately knew I had broken my leg. As soon as I could catch my breath from the immediate pain, I literally scooped up my leg with my right arm, making sure I kept it straight, and heard a grinding noise inside. I also noticed that my foot was unresponsive.

I shuffled down the remaining steps, asked one of my children to bring me my phone, called my husband and my brother-in-law (to ask him to come over to be with my kids), and then I called an ambulance.

First aid

The paramedics were with me within eight minutes, but it took them over an hour to move me out of the house and into the ambulance. I don't recall much from that hour. I remember them cutting my socks and my trousers off to get access to the leg and being particularly worried about the lack of sensitivity in my foot.

They took great care with my leg and foot, of course, making sure the limb was kept straight and supported as much as possible to minimise movement and prevent any bones from breaking through the skin. I was pretty sure my leg was broken, and from what I had told them and what they could see they agreed with me, but it's not up to the paramedics to make a diagnosis. They took my blood pressure several times and gave me morphine before they immobilised my leg and secured me onto a stretcher to put me into the ambulance.

At the hospital

When we arrived I was wheeled into the X-ray room. Moving between the hospital wheel bed and the X-ray table wasn't the easiest of tasks at that point, and moving my leg to the side so they could get the views they needed was extremely painful. In these cases, having an X-ray technician who is both experienced and empathetic makes a huge difference!

After having the X-rays done I was informed that I had broken both my tibia and my fibula. I had a stable, closed, spiral fracture on my tibial shaft, and while the doctors didn't seem worried about the fibula, they informed me straight away that I'd need surgery on my tibia. A doctor came to explain what the surgery entailed and I signed some papers to agree to it. In hindsight, this wasn't the best time to sign anything as I didn't ask any questions or read any of the small print, so don't do what I did! I wasn't even aware of the option to 'do nothing' and keep a plaster cast for six months until a few minutes before my surgery was due to start.

The doctors also informed me that because the surgery couldn't take place on that day, I'd need a temporary plaster cast (a back slab), and I'd be admitted to the hospital until after the surgery.

Having a plaster cast made while you've just broken your leg isn't the best of experiences. Just before the procedure I was offered paracetamol and codeine, and I was asked to use Entonox (also known as 'gas and air') for pain relief while the bandages were being applied. The fracture on my tibia was quite low, but my fibula was fractured at the top, so they had to immobilise my perfectly fine knee as well.

Hospital stay

I'll spare you the details of my various attempts at using the toilet while being bedridden. Let's just say that I experimented with a bedpan as well as a commode chair with various degrees of difficulty and success. An above-the-knee plaster cast is quite heavy to handle and move on your own, especially when you try to lift it yourself. You end up putting strain on your broken bone, and that's not a nice sensation! Needless to say, I did require a great deal of help from the nurses when getting changed or using the toilet at first.

I ended up waiting nearly three days for my surgery. Every day I was kept fasting (nil by mouth) until about 3.00pm. At that point when it became clear that the surgery wouldn't happen on that day, I'd be offered a late lunch. I was fed through an IV drip when I couldn't eat, and of course the nurses were in and out all day taking my temperature and measuring my blood pressure, as well as offering medication to deal with the pain. In order to minimise the risk of blood clots, I was asked to wear a compression sock on my left ('good') leg.

Surgery

I had my surgery on Sunday 4 September 2016. The orthopaedic team inserted an intramedullary nail into my right tibia with four interlocking screws (two at the top and two at the bottom). I was unconscious (under anaesthetics) for about three hours, but I doubt the surgery lasted that long.

When I woke up, I had no plaster cast but there was a bandage wrapped around my right leg, covering the knee and ankle. I was in slight discomfort, but felt relieved that everything had gone well. I was provided with a morphine drip that I could self-manage, and I was also informed I was still under the partial effect of the anaesthetic drugs, so my pain was numbed for a little longer.

I felt okay after the surgery, but also very tired. Between the pain in my leg and the fact I couldn't really turn over in bed, I found it hard to rest at night, but thanks to the residual drugs in my body and the morphine I was taking, the night after the surgery is probably the one I managed to rest the most.

Post-surgery

After my surgery, I stayed in hospital for another 48 hours. As the effects of the anaesthetic started to wear off the discomfort became more intense. Unfortunately, miscommunication between the pain management doctor and nurses looking after me meant that I wasn't given any morphine on the second night after my surgery, so I got no sleep due to the pain I was experiencing.

Among all the painkillers I was also offered some antibiotics to try to prevent the onset of infection. They were injected intravenously once a day for three days through the IV drip I had in my left hand. While I felt the liquid being pushed through during the first injection, it wasn't painful (because I was still partially under the effects of the anaesthetic), but the injections on the following days were really uncomfortable.

The day after the surgery, I was visited by a physiotherapist who provided me with a pair of elbow crutches and taught me how to use them. She showed me how to safely get out of bed and up from a chair, how to walk and how to sit down, etc. The physiotherapist's role is to make sure you can safely handle yourself and go about your daily life on crutches, and in the UK they will not give you the all-clear to be discharged unless you can safely go up and down stairs. Being near a staircase was literally the last thing I wanted to do at this point, but with a sick feeling in my stomach, I had to go up and down them on my crutches (with the help of two physiotherapists). With that all done, it meant that two days after the surgery I could be discharged.

Being discharged

Before I was sent home, the nurse came to change my bandage so I got to see my leg and the dressing for the first time. She changed the dressings over the knee incision and over the four smaller incisions made for the four interlocking screws. She also provided me with spare dressings to take to my GP so I could get those changed.

The nurse provided me with paracetamol and codeine to take home and showed my husband how to perform a heparin injection in my stomach – heparin is the anticoagulant we discussed in section 3 that helps prevent the formation of blood clots. I had to have daily injections for two weeks following my surgery.

Before we left the hospital the Occupational Therapy team were also able to provide me with a raised toilet seat, a toilet frame and an adjustable-height chair that I could use in the shower.

The first few days at home

Back at home, those early days were quite odd and difficult in a way. I have three young children (my youngest was two years old at the time), and I felt quite vulnerable without a plaster cast. I had to keep my leg elevated and that often meant it was 'in the way' (not where you'd normally find a leg when someone is sitting down), and it was quite easy for people to bash into it.

I was feeling drowsy and exhausted from the combination of having recently been under general anaesthetic, taking a considerable amount of drugs I wasn't used to and not sleeping much at night. Having been bedridden for six days by now I was also quite weak. I felt dizzy when getting up, and that didn't help at the time, seeing that I was also trying to re-train my body to walk on crutches without putting any weight on my right leg (I was light-touch weight-bearing but trying to be non-weight-bearing for the first six weeks).

The adjustments to my downstairs toilet were a lifesaver. I really appreciated the toilet frame and raised toilet seat, as well as the adjustable-height chair I used in the shower. I had to buy a waterproof leg cover to use for the first few days and weeks while my dressing was still on, as I couldn't get my leg wet. Getting in and out of the shower was also a bit of an ordeal at first, as I have a raised step to get into it, and at first I found that quite hard. Not to mention that I often felt faint when walking.

Needless to say, I did require a bit of help for the first week. I wasn't quite myself at all. And having to get used to crutches and re-train your body to do the simplest things is tricky at first. But things do get better after the first week or so!

Personally, I was keen to avoid the stairs at home – in fact I couldn't even look at them as they reminded me of the accident – so for the first couple of weeks I decided to sleep downstairs on a sofa bed. I did that until my back started screaming for mercy. Sleeping continued to be quite tricky in the first week or so after surgery. I had my leg propped up on a pillow, and I couldn't really move it to the side unless I was manually and carefully changing its position. So I was forced to sleep on my back most of the time, which I don't find comfortable and I really did struggle with sleep and rest.

Recovering

After the initial couple of weeks, I started to feel a lot stronger. I managed to rest and sleep, the pain wasn't as intense and I stopped taking medication. I didn't experience a painful rush of blood to my leg every time I got up, I started to feel less dizzy, less light-headed and faint, and I started gaining confidence on my crutches.

In short, I got used to it. You get used to moving around the house on crutches, not having the use of your hands for carrying things and having a non-weight-bearing leg. I bought non-slip socks for my left foot to ensure I had a good grip on the floor, I had a box with medications and supplements to keep by the side of the sofa (and sofa bed initially) and I had a backpack with my change of clothes or anything I needed to carry in and out of the bathroom.

I still needed help with the running of the house and managing the children of course, but over time I found my way around things, including doing the laundry and carrying small things up and down the stairs by 'bum-shuffling' on them. That's definitely not what the physiotherapist had taught me, but it worked for me and it felt a lot safer than doing the stairs with two crutches in the way without being able to put any weight on my leg. I promise I tried, but the induced anxiety (and probably panic of being on the stairs) wasn't worth the risk.

My GP changed my dressing the first time, but after that I felt quite confident I could do it by myself. After a couple of weeks or so, the wounds had started healing and I felt that the dressing wasn't really required anymore. My leg was of course bruised and went through all the colours of the rainbow while the blood was re-absorbed, but over time it started to look like a 'normal' leg again, albeit with a few more scars than it had before.

Now that I was feeling better, I was trying as much as I could to move and flex my toes, my knee and rotate my ankle. While my ankle was okay, my knee was very stiff and reduced in movement. The incision from the surgery obviously had an impact on that, as the skin felt tender and sore. A 5cm (2in) area of my leg was insensitive to touch, and I couldn't independently bend my big toe at all.

Follow-up appointments

By the time I went to my first follow-up appointment at the hospital six weeks after the surgery the X-rays showed partial healing, and when the specialist grasped my lower leg with both hands and started pressing on it, after my initial shock and horror I was relieved I didn't experience any pain. At that appointment, I was told that I could swim if I wanted to, I could use an exercise bike at home as long as I didn't feel any pain and I was told I could put partial weight on my leg (between 30% to 50% of my weight). His advice was to be guided by the pain.

My second follow-up appointment was eight weeks later, so 14 weeks after surgery. Between six and 14 weeks, I progressively let go of one crutch and started to experience a lot more mobility at home. I started to use the exercise bike and generally feel a lot stronger to the point where I had noticed (around 11–12 weeks after surgery) that I could take a couple of pain-free steps on my injured leg. However, I didn't want to start putting too much weight on it before I was told it was ready to do so, so I continued with partial weight bearing until my 14-week appointment.

At that appointment, I was told I could now put full weight on my leg and get rid of the crutches. However, the tibia wasn't fully healed yet so I was still not allowed to drive. Despite complaining of reduced mobility in my knee, I wasn't given any physiotherapy so I continued to exercise at home as I had been doing.

After my 14-week appointment I started to go for daily short walks outdoors without crutches to mindfully try to correct my limp. The pain in my foot, toes and the back of my leg was preventing me from walking correctly. It was only 18 weeks after my surgery that I started to walk my children to school – I didn't feel confident enough to do so before then, as my school run includes going up crowded stairs, over a bridge and down the stairs again, often carrying a sleepy pre-schooler. So I waited until I could feel it was safe for me to do it.

My last specialist appointment was 20 weeks after surgery at the end of January 2017. The X-rays showed my tibia had knitted together, so I was discharged and given the go-ahead to drive. With reduced mobility in my knee, pain under the sole of my foot and in my toes, a visible limp and unable to stand on my tiptoes or run I was finally provided with physiotherapy sessions, which I started in February 2017.

Physiotherapy

I had four appointments with the physiotherapy team between February and May 2017. At my first appointment they found that I had reduced mobility and swelling in my ankle, something I wasn't aware of. They also explained that the pain in the back of my leg was caused by my calf muscles having contracted and shortened during the period of inactivity. Over the following few weeks and months, through a combination of simple stretches and targeted muscle-strengthening exercises, I was able to eliminate the limp and reduce the pain in my leg.

At the time of writing in early 2018, I have regained full mobility in my leg. My right ankle has better mobility than my left one (due to a previous fracture of my left tibia, fibula and ankle lateral malleolus back in 1993). However, I still cannot kneel on my right knee due to the incision from the surgery, the side of my leg is still partially numb, my lower leg is very sensitive to cold and wet weather and I do experience tightening and soreness of the calf muscles or lower leg muscles some of the time.

Removing the hardware

Since being discharged back in January 2017 I returned to my local hospital in October 2017 to discuss the possibility of removing my intramedullary nail and screws. When the original surgery was performed, I was told it could be taken out after 12 months. At my 20-week appointment I was told the best time to remove the hardware was between 12 and 18 months, but the specialist at the time had no concerns with leaving the hardware in for life unless it started to cause any issues. Because I don't play any contact sports, there doesn't seem to be any rush to take the nail out. When I last saw the consultant in October 2017, I was advised to not have the surgery until two years from the initial surgery had passed. This is to ensure that my tibia is strong enough to withstand the removal of the nail. After all, there is a small risk that the tibia might fracture in the process so I was advised to wait a little longer.

15. What's next?

Leave a review and get in touch!

If you found this book useful, **please consider leaving a review on Amazon**. This will help others in the same situation find the book when they need it the most.

If you are a medical professional or someone who has found any errors or discrepancies in this book, please do get in touch. You can email me directly at sara@mindyourmamma.com. I will always strive to keep the information in this book accurate and relevant, so if you spot anything that requires changing I'd love to hear from you.

Also, if you're willing to share your story with others to reach more people, please do get in touch. I'd love to interview you, as the more we share our experiences, the more we can provide help and support to those who are going through this ordeal. You can find me in my corner of the internet – mindyourmamma.com – and on social media on Twitter, Facebook and Instagram (handle: mindyourmamma).

You can find more detailed information about my own story in the blog posts I wrote during my recovery over on my website mindyourmamma.com/broken-tibia-my-experience (or type bit.ly/2FsaZjy into your browser).

And finally, if you would like to receive a complete list of the products I mentioned in this book, please do drop me a line at sara@mindyourmamma.com or type the address bit.ly/2C2r8Ka in your browser. Once you've entered your preferred email address, you'll receive the list directly in your inbox.

Please do remember that all recommendations are made without guarantee on my part. I disclaim any liability in connection with the use of this information.

16. Glossary of terms (in alphabetical order)

Acetaminophen: medication that reduces pain and fever.

Acidic food: foods with a low pH (below 7) that cause acidity in the body. The lower the pH the more acidic the food is. Examples include lemon juice, sugar and processed foods, etc.

Acupuncture: a treatment derived from ancient Chinese medicine whereby needles are inserted at certain sites in the body for therapeutic purposes.

Adrenalin: a hormone produced by our bodies when we are scared or excited, for example, that makes our heart beat faster and gives us a boost of energy.

Anaesthetist: a medical doctor who administers **anaesthetics**.

Anaesthetics: a substance used in a medical setting (such as during surgery) to allow a patient to experience reduced levels of pain. See **general anaesthesia**.

Anticoagulants or blood thinners: medicines that help prevent **blood clots**.

Anti-embolism stockings: special stockings that reduce the risk of developing **blood clots**.

Anti-inflammatory: something that helps counteract the effects of **inflammation** in the body.

Antioxidants: foods that act as an anti-inflammatory.

Arnica or **arnica montana**: a natural substance known to have the ability to relieve aches and pains, bruising and swelling.

Ayurvedic medicine or **Ayurveda**: a medical system originating in India over 3,000 years ago and considered a type of **complementary and alternative medicine (CAM)**.

Back slab or **plaster back slab**: a cast that is used to immobilise a broken bone after a fracture has just occurred. It is a temporary cast that allows for immediate swelling of the fractured area and which is generally removed a few days after the original injury.

Blood clots or **venous thromboembolism (VTE)**: a serious, potentially fatal medical condition whereby a blockage occurs in either one of the deep veins in the body (known as DVT) or in one of the blood vessels that carry blood from the heart to the lungs (known as pulmonary embolism).

Bone fracture: a break created in a bone as a result of a blunt force trauma or impact.

Bone marrow: spongy tissue found at the centre of some bones that produces stem cells that can turn into different types of blood cells.

Cissus quadrangularis: a traditional herb known to promote joint and bone health.

Collagen: one of the main proteins in the connective tissues of the human body.

Comfrey or **comphrey** or **Symphytum**: herb known for its pain relief properties.

Commode chair: a movable toilet that does not use running water. It looks like a chair with toilet seat and bowl underneath.

Complementary and alternative medicine (CAM): a series of practices that are not part of standard medical care, such as massage, **Ayurveda, homeopathy**, etc.

Deep Vein Thrombosis (DVT): a **blood clot** that develops within a deep vein in the body, usually in the leg.

Embolism: see **blood clots**.

Entonox (also known as gas and air): see **nitrous oxide**.

Epsom salt: named after a saline spring in Epsom, Surrey, this salt is a naturally occurring pure mineral compound of magnesium and sulphate. When bathing in Epsom salt, these substances are easily absorbed by the skin.

Essential oils: aromatic compounds found in plants (for example the bark, seeds, flower and stem, etc.)

Femur: also known as the **thighbone**, this is the longest and strongest weight-bearing bone in the body.

Fibula: also known as the calf bone, it is located to the side of the **tibia** to which it is connected at the top and bottom. It is the smaller of the two bones in the lower leg and is a **non-weight-bearing** bone.

General anaesthesia: a state of controlled unconsciousness created in a medical setting (and managed by an **anaesthetist**), during which **anaesthetics** are used to send someone to sleep so that they do not experience pain during a medical procedure.

Haemorrhagic shock (also known as hypovolemic shock): a life-threatening condition occurring when someone loses more than one-fifth of their body's blood supply.

Hardware removal (HWR): the surgical removal of an intramedullary nail and/or any related screws or plates inserted to fix the fracture of a tibia (and fibula).

Healing touch therapy: a type of energy therapy where practitioners use their hands to support someone's physical, emotional, mental, and spiritual health.

Helychrisum: a natural medicinal plant used to make essential oils that are known for their **anti-inflammatory and antioxidant** properties.

Herbal medicine: a medical practice centred on the therapeutic use of active ingredients made from plant parts (such as flowers or roots, for example).

Homeopathic medicine or homeopathy: a set of treatments based on the use of highly diluted substances, also known as a type of **complementary and alternative medicine (CAM)**.

Horsetail grass or **Equisetum** or **snake grass**: a herb high in silicon.

Inflammation: our body's natural protective response, triggered when a part of the body is affected by foreign substances (such as bacteria, for example) or injured.

Intramedullary (IM) nail or rod, also referred to as an **interlocking nail** or **Küntscher nail** (named after the German surgeon Gerhard Küntscher): a metal (often titanium) rod surgically forced into the **medullary cavity** of a bone.

Intravenous (IV) rehydration: a procedure used to treat or prevent dehydration whereby a needle is inserted directly into a patient's veins (often on the back of their hand or the arm) and a saline solution is fed into it.

Light-touch weight-bearing (LTWB), also known as **touchdown weight-bearing** or **toe-touch weight-bearing**: a way of walking whereby the foot or toes of an injured leg may touch the floor to maintain balance but not to support any weight.

Lysine: an amino acid with a key role in building essential proteins in the body.

Medulla or **medullary cavity** or **marrow cavity**: the innermost or central cavity of a bone, where **bone marrow** is found.

Morphine: an **opioid** pain medication.

Nitrous oxide: an inhaled gas used as pain medication also known as Entonox or more simply 'gas and air.'

Non-healing or non-union: a situation whereby a fractured bone does not heal or re-unite correctly.

Non-weight bearing (NWB): a way of walking whereby no weight may be placed on an injured weight-bearing bone, such as the tibia or femur.

NSAIDs or non-steroidal anti-inflammatory drugs: medication used to relieve pain and fever and reduce **inflammation**.

Occupational therapy: a team of specialists that exists in UK hospitals to help patients who are experiencing difficulties to improve their ability to do everyday tasks.

Opioids or opiates: medications derived from opium and used as painkillers.

Paracetamol: a commonly used type of medication that reduces pain and fever.

Partial weight-bearing (PWB): a way of walking whereby only partial weight can be placed on an injured **weight-bearing bone**.

Patella, also known as the **kneecap**: the bone that covers and protects the knee joint.

Patellar tendon: the part of our body that attaches the bottom of our kneecap (see **patella**) to the top of our **tibia** (or shinbone).

Plaster cast: a 'shell' made of plaster that helps stabilise a broken bone until healing has taken place, or in the case of most patients undergoing **tibial intramedullary nail surgery**, until surgery has been performed.

Physiotherapy: a course of treatment aimed to help restore movement and function when someone has been affected by an injury, illness or disability.

Polarity therapy: a system that integrates body work, counselling, diet, exercise and other components to encourage healing.

Qi gong or **Qigong**, **chi kung** or **chi gung**: a holistic system of coordinated body movements and posture, breathing and meditation with roots in Chinese medicine and martial arts.

Reduced range of movement: the limitation of the movement of a joint (for example the ankle or knee) whereby the joint feels painful or stiff and is not moving as much as it normally would.

Reiki: a Japanese technique used for stress reduction and relaxation that is also used to promote healing.

ROM (range of movement): referring to joints and muscles, the extent by which they are able to move. See **reduced range of movement**.

Tibia, also known as the **shinbone** or **shank bone**: the largest, strongest and only **weight-bearing bone** in our lower leg.

Tibial intramedullary nail surgery: the medical procedure required to insert an **intramedullary nail or rod** into the **medullar cavity** of a person's **tibia**.

Vibration therapy: a rehabilitation technique whereby the patient stands on a vibrating platform that sends mechanical vibration through the body. Used to stimulate muscle strength and improve circulation.

Weight-bearing bone: a bone that is responsible for carrying a person's full body weight when in motion.

X-rays: a form of electromagnetic radiation that allows for images of the inside of someone's body to be created. It is fundamental for checking the status of bones and being able to diagnose a fracture.

Zheng Gu Shui: a brand of traditional Chinese medicine liniment.

17. Internet resources (in alphabetical order, per topic)

All websites were last accessed in November and December 2017. Links have been shortened to allow you to easily type them into your browser. Over time, some of the information listed below may be subject to change. As I have no control over this content, should you come across any broken links or inconsistencies, please head over to mindyourmamma.com/broken-tibia-resources, where you will find an up-to-date version of these sources.

Acupuncture

- bit.ly/2ERU8mC
- bit.ly/2Eb8mOd

Anticoagulants – bit.ly/2EbZThY

Anti-embolism stockings – bit.ly/2nV2YaW

Antioxidants – bit.ly/1oaCD6X

Bone healing (draxe.com and betterbones.com)

- bit.ly/2EchYZ1
- bit.ly/2BkBlRd

Bone strength – bit.ly/2EcHMYX

Blood clots – bit.ly/2slqcwo

Calcium – bit.ly/2EgB4gJ

Collagen-boosting foods – bit.ly/2C6YEKW

Diet – bit.ly/2EchYZ1

Essential oils – bit.ly/2EchYZ1

Food supplements

- bit.ly/2EchYZ1
- bit.ly/2EuH3Sc

General anaesthesia – bit.ly/2FY1fcu

Homeopathic products – bit.ly/2EeG1uo

Intramedullary nailing (IM nail or rod)

- bit.ly/2GZeSt4
- bit.ly/2nNy9G4 - This website contains graphic images and is aimed at a medical audience.

Non-weight-bearing exercises – bit.ly/2Eu3w1X

Occupational Therapy – bit.ly/2FWtbNG

Omega-3 – bit.ly/2H1t9pt

Other experiences of patients with an IM nail

- bit.ly/2FsaZjy
- bit.ly/2nTcgUY
- bit.ly/2FY9KnO - You need a Facebook account to use this link and you must ask to be invited to join.

Positive mindset – bit.ly/2EdtK5z

Post-surgery – bit.ly/2Bmpz8C - This article is specific to foot and ankle surgery, but some of the considerations still apply.

Scar management (essential oils) – bit.ly/2FZJl9p

Tibia fractures

- bit.ly/2ETDuTm
- bit.ly/2FYa9GQ
- bit.ly/2moVCuI

Vibration therapy

- bit.ly/2C6Vff4
- bit.ly/2H0yv45

Vitamin B – bit.ly/2C831VT

Vitamin C – bit.ly/2EcOZZ1

Vitamin D – bit.ly/2E9YIiO

Vitamin E – bit.ly/2H2CGfG

Wound care – bit.ly/2EffkpH

X-ray – bit.ly/2ndKpPJ

Acknowledgements

I would like to take this opportunity to publicly thank all the staff (including the paramedics) at **West Middlesex University Hospital (Isleworth, UK)** for the great level of medical care I received after my injury and for fixing my leg!

And of course I would also like to thank my husband, my parents and all the family members and friends who helped and supported me and our family during my recovery. Your help and support in this journey have been crucial, so thank you!

About the author

A Business Analyst by trade, Sara Bussandri left her job in 2016 to pursue a career as a writer. As a mum of three boys based in London, she is particularly interested in parenting, self-help, self-development, mindfulness and anything that helps parents to overcome stress. Her writing has appeared in a number of publications, including The Huffington Post UK. You can find Sara over on her popular blog Mind Your Mamma (mindyourmamma.com) or connect with her on social media: Twitter, Facebook and Instagram (handle: mindyourmamma).

Made in the USA
Monee, IL
03 February 2020